Allergy Therapeutics

THIS BOOK IS DEDICATED TO
SUSAN AND BILL
WHO MADE IT POSSIBLE

The electronmicrograph on the cover shows faecal particles of a mite, Dermatophagoides pteronyssinus. *It is believed that allergens in the faecal particles are significant in producing the common house-dust allergy.*

John Clarke and Euan Tovey of the Clinical Research Centre, Harrow, Middlesex.

Allergy Therapeutics

Keith Eaton LRCP, LRCS, LRFPS
Hospital Practitioner in Allergy, Reading Hospital Group

Anne Adams SRN, NDN
Practical Work Teacher in District Nursing Studies

Janet Duberley SRN, RSCN,
DipAdv Nursing Studies
Lecturer in Nursing Studies, University of Surrey

BAILLIÈRE TINDALL · LONDON

Published by BAILLIÈRE TINDALL,
a division of Cassell Ltd,
Greycoat House, 10 Greycoat Place, London SW1P 1SB

an affiliate of
Macmillan Publishing Co. Inc.
New York

First published 1982

ISBN 0 7020 0933 4

Photoset by Bookens, Saffron Walden, Essex

Printed in Great Britain by Nene Litho
Bound by Woolnough Bookbinding Ltd.
Wellingborough, Northants.

British Library Cataloguing in Publication Data

Eaton, Keith
  Allergy therapeutics.
  1. Allergy
  I. Title II. Adams, Anne
  III. Duberley, Janet
  616.97   RC584
  ISBN 0-7020-0933-4

Contents

Preface

The authors have, for some years now, been involved in providing education in the field of allergy, first for nurses and more recently for doctors and technicians. Although there are a number of large and exceedingly comprehensive books on the subject, this book has grown out of our conviction that there is a place for a short, simple and basic text to provide a groundwork that could be used both by doctors working in general practice and assisting in allergy clinics and by nurses and technicians involved in this work.

A number of developments in allergy have, in recent years, broadened the concepts involved and an increasing number of hospitals and general practitioners are now providing such services; in most general practices nurses are involved in giving hyposensitizing courses to patients. The number of people in the UK who have experienced allergic diseases is now, according to the most recent assessment, about 30% of the whole population. Not all will require specific treatment from an allergy clinic, but many will. In spite of this, the amount of instruction given to health workers in this subject, either before or after training, is minimal and it is hoped that this book will help in a small way to supply some of that need.

It is intended that it should be simple to refer to, so that it can be used in the clinic, if required, so that specific points can be easily looked up.

March 1982   Keith Eaton
Anne Adams
Janet Duberley

Acknowledgements

The illustrations on pp. 21 and 80 are reproduced by kind permission of E. Merck Ltd. For the pollination chart on p. 41 we are indebted to Dr R.R. Davies of the Department of Bacteriology, St Mary's Hospital Medical School, London. Permission to use the illustrations of skin testing technique on p. 50 were kindly provided by the Photographic Department, Royal Berkshire Hospital, Reading. The illustrations on pp. 58 and 59 are reproduced by kind permission of Pharmacia Ltd and that on p. 66 by kind permission of Dr Robert Davies of the Chest Department, St Bartholomew's Hospital.

We are indebted to Mr R.M. Auld of E. Merck Ltd for allowing us to use material which first appeared in *Practical Allergy Using Norisen Extracts* and who, by asking us to lecture on courses on allergy for nurses, first stimulated us to write this book.

We would also like to acknowledge the help and support of professional colleagues at work, without whose support and tolerance this work could never have been completed. Finally we must express our deep gratitude to Mrs Joan Barron for secretarial assistance beyond the call of duty in preparing the typescript of this book.

1

The History of Allergy

It may seem inappropriate to commence what is intended to be
a practical handbook with a chapter on the history of the
subject, but to the authors this approach seems totally defensible, on two counts. Firstly it places our present state of
knowledge in a different perspective. We know, perhaps, more
than our forebears, but less than our successors. The realization
of what has gone before increases our respect for those whose
original thinking enables us to do what we can now do, and at
the same time should prevent us from being complacent, as our
best efforts will, in due course, seem as primitive as theirs.
Secondly the names of the founding fathers in any specialty
crop up in all sorts of ways in the day-to-day work of the subject
and it is of value to know who they were and what they did.

At some point in historical time, therefore, there must be a
start. Asthma and eczema have been known since ancient times
and are described by Hippocrates and other ancient authors;
references continue through the literature of the renaissance
to the eighteenth century and so to modern times. However,
the link with allergy is a recent connection. By contrast, hay
fever does not feature in the writings of the ancients; indeed the
first medical report on the subject does not occur until the early
nineteenth century. Under such circumstances we sometimes
find that references which are absent in the scientific literature
can be found in lay publications and the works of great writers
have always been a fruitful field for this. In this case, however,
no early reports can be found by such search and so we come up
to the year of 1819 when John Bostock read a paper which was
published in the *Medico-Chirurgical Transactions of London*, in that
year. It was entitled 'Case of a Periodical Affection of the Eyes
and Chest' and was an account of one single case of this new
disease. The author, a London physician, had no difficulty in

maintaining contact with this interesting medical curiosity, for the patient was himself. However, he pursued a keen interest in the subject, and nine years later in 1828 was able to report that he had either seen or received 'distinct accounts of eighteen cases', together with about ten others less well documented. This gives an incidence for a doctor obviously keenly interested in the condition of three cases a year. Obviously since this early stage hay fever has become very much more common and this difference in incidence cannot be attributed solely to under-reporting. Now we find allergy in perhaps 30% of the total population and a general practitioner may see five or ten cases a day in the peak month of June. In the allergy clinic run by one of the authors an average new case referral rate at peak times of year is 30, with perhaps the same number again of follow-up patients.

From 1828 hay fever no longer languished without documentation. Bostock considered the case of 'hay asthma' to be heat, but Gordon, writing in 1829, attributed the blame to 'the aroma emitted by the flowers of grass'. At the time his voice went largely unheeded, for it was Bostock's view which generally gained acceptance, and this view was keenly reinforced by the work of von Philipp, Professor of Medicine at Geissen, who in 1859 produced what was then the definitive work on the subject. His results were really a very early example of research by questionnaire (today a very fashionable research tool), as he obtained his statistics by correspondence with doctors in various countries and confined his own efforts to collation of the results. He surveyed various headings, geographical distribution (the disease was then most common in England), whether or not it affected foreigners as well as natives, sex distribution, social class (most common in the educated classes in England, a difference less common on the Continent), genetic predisposition, family history, concomitant disease and time of year.

An increasing number of papers now appeared on the subject, but none of them appear to shed any new light. For this we must move forward to the year 1873 and the work of Charles Harrison Blackley, a Manchester homeopathic physician, who then published the classic book *Experimental Researches on the*

Cause and Nature of Catarrhus Aestivus (Hay Fever or Hay Asthma). This book still serves today as an example of how one man can change the face of a subject without outside assistance. He reviewed all the literature and from this obtained a list of suggested causes. A sufferer himself, he was then able to put each individual theory to the test by trying out each suggestion. These included benzoic acid, perfumes and odours, ozone, heat and light. These did not produce the symptoms. However, dust from the side of a road in the hay fever season did, but he found that it contained grass pollen. Taking grass pollen alone, he succeeded in inducing experimental hay fever. Using his microscope he identified numerous pollens and measured their effects on himself by instilling them into his eyes and nose and inhaling them into his lungs. By these means he showed that only pollens could be relied upon to produce symptoms in the winter as well as the summer. He must have been a highly sensitized subject, as he reacted to the pollens of grasses, cereals, garden and wild flowers, weeds, trees and some species that even he could not identify. One species caused what we now know as a delayed reaction which he clearly documents. He found pollens to be seasonally present in the air and devised the first spore trap by which he was able to measure the world's first pollen counts. Those for the period of May to August 1866 appear in his book. As now, the peak was in the month of June at the peak of the hay fever season. He flew a kite and collected pollen at altitude, showing that it rises with the warm currents of air. Sadly he was less successful in treatment and the best he could devise, after many trials, was to advise 'a cruise in a yacht, which can be kept well out to sea . . . or failing this a sojourn on a small island in the open ocean'.

The term **allergy** was first used by the German pathologist Clemens Peter von Pirquet in 1906. The term means 'altered in reaction' and comes from the Greek *allos* (altered) and *ergon* (reaction). He states that 'The vaccinated person behaves in a different manner from him who has not previously been in contact with such an agent, yet he is not insensitive to it. So we can say of him that his power to react has undergone a change. For this general concept of change I propose the term "allergy".'

In 1911 a young surgeon, Leonard Noon, was researching in

the Wright Fleming Institute of St Mary's Hospital in London. Originally looking at bacteria, he turned to hay fever and discovered that serial injections of grass pollen dissolved in water would lessen the severity of the attack. His method was published in the *Lancet* in June of that year. In addition to devising an effective course of anti-allergic treatment for grass pollen sufferers, he also laid down the first unit of allergic activity still in use today and known as the Noon unit. From this commencement, a good deal of refining has taken place and the preparation of dosage level of our courses given today owe much to the detailed work of his successors at St Mary's Hospital, especially Dr Freeman and Dr A.W. Frankland, who established this as one of the leading allergy units of the world.

From this point on the emphasis changes; work has turned to establishing the mechanisms which cause the reaction. In 1923 two Americans, Coca and Cooke, referred to the hereditary aspects and the differences between the allergic and non-allergic populations. They described the reaction by a term which means 'out of place', **atopy**. The most important discovery in our understanding of the mechanisms controlling the production of allergy was the discovery of immunoglobulin E (IgE), which was the work of Ishizaka and his colleagues, not published till 1966. This substance will be more fully discussed in Chapter 3.

In addition to treatment by desensitization, we are all familiar with palliative treatment with antihistamines. This important group of drugs derives from experimental work in France just before the First World War, but the first effective drug for human use did not appear until 1942, in France; its final form was mepyramine maleate, which was first put on the market in 1944 as Neo-Antergan, known in Great Britain as Anthisan. In the United States, because of the breakdown in scientific communication caused by World War II, parallel work had continued with the original 1937 compound; this led to the introduction in 1946 of diphenhydramine (Benadryl), which was also the first antihistamine in Britain in the same year. Since then a vast number of alternative formulations have appeared.

The other most significant palliative has emerged more

recently. Disodium cromoglycate was first made available in 1967 following the work of Altounyan, one of the latest to use himself as his own experimental subject.

Upon this note we may conclude this chapter, with the realization that after 150 years of allergy research we still find that a significant and important place remains for those who use themselves as their own guinea-pigs for research. It is worth remembering that as allergists we shall have few guinea-pigs referred to us for treatment—but an awful lot of people!

2

Allergy and Allergens

Up to now we have considered the subject in general terms, but to come to grips with it we must become more precise. The first step is to define what we mean by the various technical terms that are used to provide the basic scientific vocabulary necessary to discuss the condition. As we have seen in Chapter 1 the term allergy is relatively new—and yet it has got into the popular vocabulary of the lay public. Whenever this happens the meaning of the word becomes changed and distorted. As professionals we must be careful to ensure that when we use such words we do not accept the inexact 'public' meaning, but stick to the correct one at all times.

ALLERGY is defined as an abnormal, altered and specific sensitivity to a particular substance or substances known as allergens. Let us see what this means. Firstly, the reaction is *abnormal*. Most people do not react in this way, only a proportion of the population. One of the authors intermittently experiences allergic symptons, the others never have. Secondly, the reaction is *altered*. Contrary to public belief, no one is 'born with allergy'. It is always acquired. Thirdly, allergy is *specific*. Every human is exposed to hundreds, if not thousands, of substances by which an allergy can be induced. Few people, even the most severely troubled, are sensitive to more than a handful. Most are allergic to one or two only. The reaction can be specific even within the substance involved. A patient with hay fever may be allergic to one particular grass pollen and not to others, or an asthmatic to one cat and not to another. Fourthly, allergy is a *sensitivity*, which implies that the problem is present in dilution. Almost anyone who decides to sweep out an attic where the dust has been undisturbed for over a hundred years will probably sneeze. This is irritation, exactly as when inhaling pepper, and not allergy. It becomes an allergy when the problem will occur in response to the agent in dilution: a dust-sensitive patient may sneeze even when sleeping on a bed where the mattress is vacuumed each day.

The substances causing these reactions are known as allergens.

Allergens are defined as the substances identified as causing allergic reactions. They are generally proteins, but can be glycoproteins (proteins with a glycogen or carbohydrate fraction in the molecule) or *haptens*. The latter are chemical substances which do not truly become allergenic until they combine with protein, usually within the body. This group is now beginning to assume an increasing importance because of industrial sources of such substances. Simple metals such as copper can by haptens. We have all seen the greenish stain on the skin occasionally produced by a copper bracelet for 'rheumatism'. Newer substances such as platinates are not protein and, therefore, one presumes are allergens because they behave as haptens.

In allergy a number of synonyms are used. Thus, as an alternative to the term allergy, the term **atopy** is sometimes used. Originally coined by Coca, it actually means 'a strange state'. At various times individual writers have sought to invest the word with a specific and separate meaning of its own, but none of these has gained universal acceptance. The term **atopic** (one who suffers from atopy) is used in much the same way that physicians refer to neoplasm rather than cancer. It provides a private language that the patient cannot share. Its use in this way is to be deprecated; indeed, in logical terms it is difficult to see the need for two terms for the same condition, provided that one is used correctly.

The term **antigen** used as a synonym for allergen is more defensible, because this word derives from basic immunology (see Chapter 3) and at first sight seems an attractive alternative. However, an antigen–antibody reaction takes place with a much wider range of substances than the allergens and normally results in an immune rather than a hypersensitive response, whereas the allergen induces the opposite effect. When we use the term antigen we are not specifying whether the response will be immunity or hypersensitivity; when we use the term allergen we are. Technically, antigen is formed when the allergen or hapten combines with tissue protein.

To sum up, allergy has a few terms which are all its own. Correctly used they aid communication between those working on the subject. Incorrectly used they cause confusion and may even lead to mistakes involving patient care. Be sure always, therefore, to use these words, as with all medical terms, with an acute awareness of their true meaning.

Having now covered the basic language we are going to employ, we must examine the basic reaction with which the whole subject is concerned. The immunological basis of the response will be found in Chapter 3, but the clinical aspects fall in this chapter.

THE ALLERGIC REACTION

Allergic reactions take place at points of contact between the body and the outside world.

Thus the *eyes* and the lining of the *nose* and *throat* are exposed to air which contains allergens in profusion, and typically a reaction involving all these 'target organs' is present in hay fever and in perennial rhinitis. The eyes may react on their own and the condition is then often called vernal conjunctivitis or spring catarrh. Allergic conjunctivitis may be a better term, as the other implies that the condition only occurs in spring and is seasonal. For many sufferers this is not so.

The lining of the *lungs* is, of course, also exposed to contact with the air and the contents of the air, and manifests its reaction in the form of asthma.

The *skin* covering the whole of the body is clearly exposed to insult from the outside world, although partially protected by its keratinized outer layers, and may respond by eczema, urticaria or angio-oedema.

Finally, the *gut*, as a hollow tube passing through the body, is exposed to foreign material passing through and may respond by developing symptoms.

Until the advent of modern medicine these were the only surfaces exposed to contact with outside agents, but it is now possible by injection or transfusion to introduce such factors into the veins or tissues anywhere in the body. This may give rise to a new complex of allergies such as serum sickness. These will be mentioned for completeness, but do not normally fall within the province of the allergist.

Hay fever

Hay fever is defined as a seasonal affliction of the eyes, nose, throat and lungs. Any or all may be involved. Classical hay fever is a response to grass pollen and takes place in the grass pollen season; in Great Britain this is usually June and early July. The term is extended to cover other pollen responses which may occur between February and August.

The symptoms are governed by the pathological reactions taking place. Let us remind ourselves what they are. Sequential reactions take place at a mucosal surface. They are *irritation, secretion* and *oedema*. Hay fever is no exception in this respect and to regard the reactions in this way helps our understanding of the symptoms and creates a logical sequence. The initial response is irritation and the irritated eye responds by becoming red and by itching. The irritated nose responds by itching and sneezing and the irritated chest gives a dry non-productive cough. Secretion follows next. The eyes water and the nose runs. Both these discharges are clear and not coloured. Down in the lung the position is less easy to identify, but the cough becomes productive and the secretions in the narrow bronchi cause diminished airflow which produces the audible wheezing we all know as bronchospasm. In the past the term rhonchi has been used for this condition, but this term has been defined in different ways and it is now thought that wheeze is better and less subject to error. The final response is oedema. In the eyes this is marked by swelling of the sclera, which by this time is usually so infected as to be blood-red all over and exuding a yellowish gelatinous material. The cornea remains clear, so vision is not affected. Swelling of the eyelids or blepharitis may also occur. In severe allergic conjunctivitis the conjunctiva becomes red and swollen and develops 'cobblestone' papillae which may rub on the cornea. Again there is a thick discharge which is sometimes described as ropy.

Both these conditions, having reached the stage of oedema,

are to be regarded as emergencies requiring prompt treatment; if they remain untreated, ulceration may occur and vision may thus be affected, sometimes with permanent loss of sight. In the nose oedema gives rise to nasal obstruction and in the chest oedema increases the severity of the wheeze and lessens the ability to cough up sputum. The term *pollenosis* is often used to describe the sum of these manifestations.

Vernal conjunctivitis (spring catarrh)

Vernal conjunctivitis or spring catarrh is defined as a seasonal or non-seasonal ophthalmic reaction to an allergen. Very often it does occur in spring, as the name suggests, any time from February to April or May; in this form it is usually associated with tree pollens. However, as we have seen above, the condition may occur with grass pollen and it may also occur with perennial allergens. Thus the name is not a good one. Nevertheless as it has stood the test of time it remains in use; although it would be easy to propose an alternative, such a name should have universal acceptance. There have been too many names for conditions which lack this essential prerequisite. The symptoms are as discussed above in hay fever.

Asthma

Asthma is defined as variation in airways resistance. This is a cumbersome definition and not easy of access. The problem with asthma is that, although it appears easy to recognize clinically, the variations of presentation are extreme and it is difficult to find a definition which covers them all. Extensive discussions have led to a formula which covers the main measurable factor which can be objectively determined. In asthma the breathing capacity is reduced during attacks, but improves and may even return to normal in between. However, in chronic bronchitis, although the breathing capacity is reduced, the reduction is constant and does not vary significantly from day to day, from week to week, or even from month to month.

This breathing capacity can be measured using a variety of spirometric devices. The best measure is the total lung volume and the rate at which the patient can attain this total. Instruments are available which give a digital read-out measured electronically, but these are expensive and hence rare. The Vitalograph, however, is a standard machine which is available in many clinics and gives a ready measurement of *forced vital capacity* (FVC), defined as the gas volume expired after maximum inspiration, with expiration being as rapid and complete as possible, i.e. forceful. The *forced expiratory volume* (FEV) is defined as the gas volume expired over a given time interval during a forced expiration following a maximum inspiration. The FEV time usually taken is one second, the measurement then being known as FEV_1. There are a number of other measurements that can be taken with this machine, but these are the ones in common use. Although this machine is simple to use an even simpler device is the peak flow meter, which measures the *peak expiratory flow* (PEF) defined as the maximum rate of air flow obtained on a forced expiration after a maximum inspiration. This machines comes in two sizes, standard and low-reading for patients with a PEF of below 200. Even cheaper versions of this instrument, called peak flow gauges, are produced at a price so low that no clinic, however, poor, need or should be without one. Examples are shown of serial peak flow readings on patients showing how those of a patient with asthma vary and those of one with bronchitis do not (see illustration p. 68). It should be noted that as a cheaper instrument, the peak flow gauge, does not retain its accuracy indefinitely and should be checked from time to time against a standard meter or replaced.

Eczema

Eczema is defined as a tissue reaction involving the epidermis and upper portion of the dermis, brought about by the action on these areas of substances to which the skin is allergic. The appearances vary widely. There may be vesicular eruptions or a dull red glazed erythematous response. This may be followed by skin cracking and an exudative phase. As the reaction progresses, scaling or lichenification may appear. The response may be flexural, generalized or localized. The skin is not a mucous membrane and therefore the reactions seen are not as simple to observe as in the eyes, nose or lung, but from the description given it will be seen that an element of parallel responsiveness is present.

Urticaria ('hives', nettle rash)

Urticaria is defined as multiple raised, markedly irritant (itching) skin lesions, each displaying the classical triple response of red line, flare and weal. These are clearly seen. The lesions may be vesicular and may weep. This rash in its acute form is the classical 'allergy rash' known to the general public and diagnosed by most doctors and nurses as being of allergic origin. This may be true of acute urticaria, although many cases lack any traceable cause, but is certainly not true of chronic urticaria. This may even be a different condition and patients attending dermatologists or allergists in the United Kingdom are found to have an identifiable cause (not always allergic) in only about 10% of the cases evaluated.

Angio-oedema (angioneurotic oedema)

Angio-oedema is defined as an acute local oedema of the skin. It may accompany urticaria. It is usually present in the region of the mouth, eyelids and cheeks, but may extend to the neck, pharynx, tongue and glottis, where respiratory obstruction may result in a fatal asphyxia. In this severe form it is the least common allergic response, but in milder forms it is a very common experience and is frequently seen by general practitioners, although only the more severe forms need hospital referral.

Food allergy

No consideration of allergy at the present time would be complete without an attempt to evaluate food allergy, or food intolerance as some consider it should be designated. The subject is not new in concept; we are all familiar with the urticarial rash which may follow the ingestion of, for example, strawberries. This may properly be listed under the differential diagnosis of urticaria and does not merit a section on its own.

The current view of food sensitivity arises from the fact that many patients investigated for this condition show evidence of *multiple allergy*. We frequently see this in simple hay fever where the patient may exhibit reactivity to pollens other than grass and may respond in the season to such things as animal danders, which do not bother him at other times. Thus there are several simultaneous allergies which cannot be validly diagnosed or treated in isolation. It is only since a method which permits identification of several allergenic foods has been developed that the commonness of the syndrome has been grasped.

An equally relevant factor is that of *non-immediate reactivity*. This will be fully discussed in Chapter 3 and therefore at this stage it must suffice to state that many of the reactions to foods do not take place, as does the rash after strawberries, with a rapid onset which enables both patient and doctor to pinpoint it by simple observation.

From the foregoing it may be surmised that many of the advances which are now being made in this field have come about as a result of the evaluation of the diagnostic process which is used. The role of different modes of testing, such as skin tests, will be found in Chapter 6 and laboratory tests in Chapter 7. The technique which has led to these discoveries is *elimination dieting* and will be discussed in Chapter 8.

Many patients referred for assessment in the allergy clinic tend to have additional problems, often of long standing, in addition to the presenting condition which has caused their referral. Some of these are clearly allergic conditions, but many appear not to be. Of course we are used to the fact that many people will have had several of the common diseases and that those which tend to chronicity may still be with them. It is thus no surprise to find that a patient may have had, for example, cystitis, as it is a very common condition. Where we should take notice is when patients with the same grouping of symptoms report in a particular clinic and report that treatment for one condition has ameliorated all their other ills. This not infrequently seems to be the case in food sensitivity. The authors therefore propose the term the *food allergy syndrome* to cover such responses. The common symptoms normally do not relate to only one organ system and no logical connecting thread appears in the absence of food sensitivity. The absence of some symptoms is not evidence that the condition is not present, nor without confirmation will the presence of all of them be incontravertable proof that food allergy is the correct diagnosis. In the authors' opinion the presence of several of the symptoms listed below always makes an investigation for food allergy warrantable. Such an investigation is extremely cheap to undertake and, under proper supervision, devoid of significant risk to the patient. The same is clearly not true of some of the many tests which may be engendered if food allergy is not present. Such investigations will, of course, have been negative if the true diagnosis is food sensitivity. The list does not attempt to be exhaustive, but is an attempt to indicate the commonest reported occurences.

Medications

Finally, in the catalogue of the manifestations of allergy, we should consider the effects of introducing medications into the body. These include *drug hypersensitivity reactions, transfusion reactions* and *serum sickness*. Such conditions are obviously normally dealt with by the physicians or surgeons concerned and do not fall within the province of the allergist, although occasionally an immunologist may be involved in diagnosing the precise cause of the patient's reactivity.

THE RESULTS OF ALLERGY

The last aspects we will consider in this chapter are the general and social consequences of allergy to the community. Many of the commonest manifestations of allergy are seasonal and the season coincides with the timing of all of the most important examinations for young people—and, of course, allergies are largely diseases of young people. CSE examinations, O levels,

Symptoms which may indicate food allergy

Ophthalmic	Conjunctivitis
	Blepharitis
ENT	Rhinitis
	Eustachian tube obstruction
	Sinus pain
	Oral reactions (pain, tingling, oedema, apthous ulcers)
Chest	Asthma
	Idiopathic bronchorrhoea
Skin	Pruritus
	Eczematous rashes
	Urticarial rashes
Gastrointestinal	Nausea and/or vomiting
	Abdominal pain
	Constipation
	Diarrhoea
	'Spastic colon'
Cardiac	Tachycardia
	Palpitations
	Non-anginal chest pain
Genitourinary	Frequency
	Dysuria
	Vaginal discharge
Psychiatric	Anxiety
	Depression
	Obsessional states
Neurological	Headache
	Migraine
	Muscular weakness
	Reduced concentration
	Blurred vision
	Paraesthesiae
	Reduction in perception of printed texts
Locomotor	Joint pain and/or swelling
	'Fibrositis'

A levels, City and Guilds examinations and university degree examinations all coincide with the hay fever season. This may result in candidates doing less well than they should and may even permanently block career prospects. Asthma produces intermittent illness necessitating time off school and work, which may result in failure to progress or loss of job. Both may result in the victim slipping down the social scale and ending up in the poorer section of the community. The skin manifestations are unsightly and may limit job prospects: society places a premium on looking good. Lastly asthma and angio-oedema may be fatal, with consequences not only for the patient but also for his or her family. We must always remember these broader aspects of the work that we undertake, for this work is concerned with people.

3

The Immunological Basis of Allergy

Allergy as a specialty has a very close relationship with the growing science of immunology. Although, undoubtedly, the allergists have acted as a spur to the immunologists in making progress, the subject is now so well established that the laboratory discoveries of academic immunology are flooding in upon the clinical workers, providing a whole new foundation upon which we must base our practices, which may have to be modified in the light of new knowledge.

THE IMMUNE SYSTEM

Immunology is the science of the processes and factors which protect the body against invasion by foreign material.

Non-specific immunity is present in all species and represents a general line of defence. Certain conditions are species-specific. For example, a human may safely handle a rabbit which has died from myxomatosis, without fear of contracting the disease. Man has a species immunity to this virus. By contrast, a rabbit which does not contract the condition when exposed has a specific immune response. A number of factors contribute to non-specific immunity, including hormones, enzymes, macrophages and polymorphonuclear white blood cells. All of these will react to any foreign material entering the body, but are unable to distinguish between one source of material and another. The macrophage, a silk suture and a smallpox virus are of interest—but the interest is equal.

Specific immunity is a more valuable protection because it enables the body to produce a greater effort to contend against more significant intruders. Such specific immunity depends upon *recognition*. In order to recognize and respond to any substance, the body must have met it before. On the first occasion it is identified and therefore when the same substance is met again recognition is immediate; it is this recognition which leads to the response. *Passive* specific immunity is gaining an increasing importance in allergy, because antibodies to a number of substances are transferred across the placenta and through breast milk. This process protects the newborn baby to some extent and the fact that the baby is not receiving the potentially sensitizing cows milk may avoid premature exposure before its own antibody system has begun to work. The latter is considered important in the onset of infantile eczema and this may be relevant in the later development of hay fever and asthma. *Active* specific immunity is produced by disease or immunization. The process is the same in conditions like poliomyelitis, caused by a virus, with immunization being affected by a weakened live virus, or in tetanus, a bacterial infection where a killed vaccine is used.

Two separate chains of reactivity exist. The **humoral** or endocrine chain causes the release of free antibody to neutralize the antigen. Mainly, however, we are concerned with the **cell-mediated** response, effected through the sensitized white cells. These are largely *lymphocytes*, although similar processes may be involved with neutrophils. Lymphocytes arise from bone marrow stem cells, but thereafter the lymphoblasts (primitive lymphocytes) are processed in areas like the lymphoid tissue of the tonsils and gut. The tissues carrying out this process are supposed to be similar to the bursa of Fabricius which is present in the chicken; the similarities in man are a postulate, but nevertheless the cells are known as the 'B' or bursa series. Immunologists frequently refer to these cells merely as T cells or B cells. The need to know of the existence of the two varieties depends upon their differing reactions when an antigen enters the body. B lymphocytes are concerned with humoral antibody mechanisms, whereas the T cells from the Thymus are concerned with cell-mediated responses. Both series of cells are required, as certain T cells react with certain B cells to produce the responses; these are known as 'helper' cells. There are also 'killer' T and B cells which are necessary to prevent the defence response itself getting out of hand. Most biological mechanisms have such a 'feedback' control to regulate the procedure.

In addition to the lymphocyte mechanism, there is *complement*. This is an enzymatic system of serum proteins which act in sequence to produce a substance which helps to dissolve the cell walls of invading cells. The sequence involved is rather like that involved in blood clotting, with several steps taking place; there are two different ways by which the end result is achieved, known as the *classical* and *alternative pathways*. In cell-mediated reactions complement is not invariably involved to a full extent. There are nine components but sometimes only four are required, as when a bacterium is engulfed by a macrophage.

Throughout this book reference has been made to antibody, but now we must consider the exact nature of the substances concerned. These are the *immunoglobulins* which are divided into five classes. The best known are IgG, IgA and IgM, which are present in blood in large amounts and are measurable in milligrams.

IgG is responsible for the immune responses to bacteria and viruses.

IgA is concerned with protection at mucosal surfaces and in the gut.

Antibodies associated with blood groups and reactions of this sort are *IgM*-mediated.

IgD and*IgE* are the remaining antibody classes. They are present in blood in very much smaller quantities than the above three and their molecular size is less. They are measured in nanograms. IgD is of concern in rheumatology, but may be a precursor of IgE.

Deficiency of one or more of these antibody systems is known to occur and when it does the resultant illness is known as **immunodeficiency**. There is a complex relationship between some of these cases of immunodeficiency and allergy.

IgE, or **reaginic antibody**, is the chief immunoglobulin class with which the allergist is concerned. Its role in normal health is not known. It is, however, markedly increased in patients with intestinal helminth infestations and may, therefore, be implicated in defence against these. However, in allergy the level of

IgE is raised and the substance is intrinsically connected with immunology of the allergic process because the molecules bind to cells called **mast cells**. Mast cells abound in the lymph nodes in the skin and in the mucosa where allergens may threaten entry to the body.

The facing illustration shows the sequence of events which takes place, a sequence known as the **anaphylactic reaction**. Upon first entry to the body of an antigen labelled 'A' it proceeds to the mast cell in the regional lymph node. The antigen provokes reactions by the T and B lymphocytes, together with complement as seen above, and IgE is formed. The IgE is attached by a portion of its molecule to the cell surface of the mast cell, which is now designated a *sensitized* mast cell, represented by a 'Y' on the diagram. No further reaction takes place at this juncture, but this is the phenomenon, discussed above, of *recognition*. Upon a second or subsequent entry of the same antigen to the body, a new reaction occurs. This time the antigen binds on to the receptor sites present on the IgE molecules on the sensitized cell, represented by ¥ on the diagram. It will be seen that this reaction is specific to the antigen 'A'. The other antigen 'D' requires a different IgE receptor site and will not bind on to one which will receive an 'A'. Thus the IgE is *specific*. The diagram also shows the internal structure of the mast cell, which will be seen to be filled with granular spots, known as *basophil granules*, because of their staining response in the laboratory. When the second reaction on the cell surface occurs, the interaction between antigen and antibody (IgE) on the cell surface causes disruption of the mast cell wall and the granules are released, causing the release of the mediators of allergy.

The best known of these **mediators** is *histamine*, but the researches of the immunologists have added a very large number of additional factors which contribute to the clinical picture. These include *SRSA* (slow-reacting substance of anaphylaxis), *serotonin, kinins, ECFA* (eosinophil chemotactic factor of anaphylaxis) and *prostaglandins* E and F. As yet there is a very limited clinical relevance for these substances, but this will undoubtedly increase as pharmacologists develop antagonists to them which can be used in treatment.

THE ALLERGIC REACTION

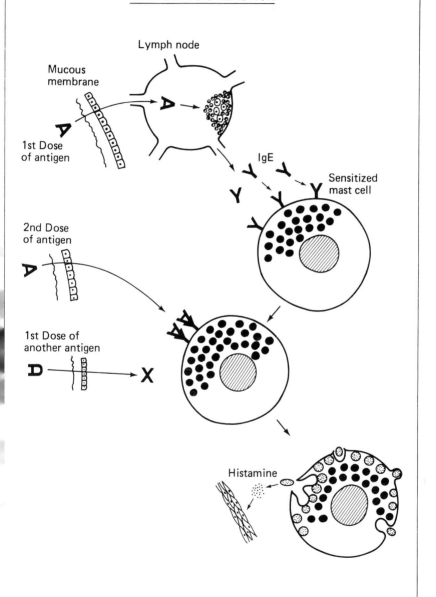

Histamine causes increased capillary permeability, vaso-dilatation and smooth muscle contraction and attracts eosino-phils. Although the inflammatory response produced by release of this material causes annoying symptoms, it does have a protective benefit for the body in confining reactivity to a local area and diminishing distant spread of an antigen throughout the system.

As yet the allergic process has been considered only in relation to the type of reactivity which occurs immediately on the entry of an antigen to the body, but for a long time it has been known that more than one type of reaction can take place to foreign invaders. The codification of this reaction by Gell and Coombs in 1963 has long been accepted as the standard comparative method and must now be considered. These authors divided reactions into four, known as **types I, II, III** and **IV reactions**. Conventionally, roman figures are always used when describing these. The table facing shows the four types and some of the clinical events in which they occur.

We have already considered type I reaction in some detail. Type II is a *cytotoxic* reaction, which means that it is present at a cell surface and results in damage to that cell. The clinical allergist will gain little experience in this type of reactivity. However, type III reactions are altogether different and have a considerable importance to the clinician. The reaction is also known as the *Arthus reaction* (pronounced 'artoos'), as it was first described by this worker, in another context. For a type III reaction to take place there must be a preceding type I reaction. The antigen and antibody, remaining locally in excess, then react together to form an insoluble complex which is tissue-damaging. For example, in farmers' lung, probably the commonest reaction where the type III response is known to occur, the patient exposed to mouldy hay may be unaware of the very minor type I reaction. However, some hours later, usually after finishing work, he develops cough, shortness of breath and sometimes pyrexia, which may persist all night. After this experience, a degree of irreversible lung damage takes place and each subsequent exposure makes this worse. Type IV reactions are, we now realize, far more common than used to be thought, but the group is so large and heterogeneous that it

Types of allergic reaction

Type I	Type II	Type III	Type IV
Immediate, anaphylactic	Cytotoxic	Antigen–antibody complex	Delayed hypersensitivity, cell-mediated
Onset within 10 minutes	Onset after several hours	Onset in four to six hours	Onset after several hours or days
Resolves in three hours	Duration 24–48 hours	Maximal at six hours; fades over next few hours	Extended duration
Examples: Hay fever Bee/wasp stings Asthma	Examples: Hypersensitivity Haemolytic disease of the newborn Transfusion reactions	Examples: Serum sickness Allergic aspergillosis Industrial inhalants Farmers' lung Asthma	Examples: Tuberculosis Contact eczema Asthma

may in due course be further subdivided. The reactions are cell-mediated. This type of reaction occurs in some inhalant allergies, but is more common in eczema and food allergies.

The remaining factor in an evaluation of the immunology of allergy concerns the mode of inheritance of allergy. From the onset of the first organ transplants it became known that transplants could be effected only between persons of like tissue make-up, as well as of like blood-group and this matching system has been resolved into a system of tissue typing known as the **HLA system**, standing for *human leucocyte antigen*. Subsequently this system has been studied in more depth and it has been found that certain HLA types are associated with certain diseases. This is true of allergy where the inheritance factors would appear to be certain of these tissue types together with a high serum IgE. This does not imply that the recipient of this genetic burden will necessarily develop allergy in a clinical way, but he is likely to pass on his own tissue types; this may serve in part to explain why allergies sometimes seem to 'skip' a generation.

Finally, it is relevant to consider in this chapter the formation of what is called **blocking antibody**. We have seen that the anaphylactic reaction is caused by the antigen reacting with IgE, followed by mast cell degranulation. This pathway is the sequence in the sensitized allergic patient, but allergens do not affect all members of the population in this way; in subjects who are not sensitive the antigen, upon entering the body, combines not with an IgE molecule, but with IgG. Under these circumstances, the IgG is known as blocking antibody because it is blocking the allergic reaction.

This concludes an account of the immunology of the allergic process. This account is necessarily both abbreviated and simplified. More information about the immune system can be found in many of the books listed under Sources of Help (p. 119). The importance of this subject ensures that with the passage of time research will teach us more about its complexities. It is a particularly rapidly developing field and the authors recommend that you should use every opportunity to keep up to date.

4

Individual Allergens

Having described the nature of the allergic process and its effects in general terms, we must consider the individual substances which can cause the complaints. No such list can ever be complete or exhaustive, as new factors are discovered each week and new industrial processes create an increasing number of man-made allergens with similar frequency. However, as in all fields of health work, most symptoms are caused by a small number of common things and the bulk of your patients should be covered by the list in this chapter.

We shall, therefore, describe in order the common allergens and their occurrence. On p. 41 we include a diagram which shows these substances represented on an annual distribution chart to enable those of you involved in history-taking to know which substances are likely to be involved at any particular time, and the time of occurrence of any allergen which the patient may consider affects him.

POLLENS

Grasses

Although there are a large number of different species of grass in the United Kingdom it is believed that only a limited number are responsible for grass pollen sensitivity. Brief botanical details of these are given below.

Bent (Agrostis tenuis). Generally distributed throughout the British Isles, mainly in acid soils such as heaths and moorland. Pollinates from June to August.

Brome (Bromus gigantum). Grows throughout the United Kingdom except for the north of Scotland, particularly in woods and shady places. Pollinates in June and July.

Cocksfoot (Dactylis glomerata). Generally distributed throughout the British Isles, particularly in waste places, fields and woods. Pollinates from early June through to September.

Dogtail (Dactylis cynosurus). Of the same family as cocksfoot and with similar distribution and pollination time. Pollinates June to August.

Fescue (Festuca eliator). Grown in meadow and grassy places throughout the British Isles though rarely found in the north of Scotland. Pollination occurs in June.

Foxtail (Alopecurus pratensis). Generally found throughout the British Isles, although more rare in Ireland. Found in damp meadows, pastures and open grassland. Pollinates from April to June.

Meadow grass (Poa pratensis). Commonly occurs throughout Europe in meadows, grassy places and on dunes. Pollination occurs in May, June and July.

Rye grass (Lolium perenne). While sometimes sown for fodder it is distributed generally in the British Isles and Europe and may be found in waste places. Owing to its hard-wearing qualities it is sown on lawns, motorway verges and playing fields. Pollination commences in May and continues in June and July; there is a second pollination in August.

Timothy (Phleum pratense). Found throughout the British Isles, although rarely in the north. May be sown for hay and grass and occurs naturally in meadows. Pollination occurs in July.

Vernal (Anthoxanthum odoratum). Found throughout the British Isles on heaths and moors and in meadows and pastures. Grows on all soil types. Pollinates from April to June.

Yorkshire fog (Holcus lanatus). Grows abundantly throughout the British Isles (not only in Yorkshire) and Europe, particularly in waste places, fields and woods. Pollinates from early June through to September.

Grasses are normally tested and administered as a mixture, as patients are rarely sensitive to only one grass and cross-reactivity is common with grass allergens. Of the three firms involved in allergy manufacturing in the United Kingdom, one uses all twelve, one specifies six and one five of these individual pollens. It is possible to obtain individual extracts of single pollens, but these are rarely used except in research. 'Classical' hay fever, occurring solely in May, June and July, usually maximal towards the end of this period and well described by Frankland as 'Wimbledon fortnight reaction', is almost invariably caused by grass pollen sensitivity; only rarely is any other factor of great importance. The exception is those patients worse in wet weather and indoors in the hay fever season.

Cereals

Allergy to cereal pollens will normally be found in patients who live or work near fields of cultivated grass, for that is what cereals are, or who have contact with the seed or grain of the particular cereal. Note that cereal pollen is not the same as the grain, which is the ripened seed. Pollination obviously takes place before harvest time. Allergy to cereal pollens does not imply allergy to the processed grain or flour, nor does the reverse necessarily apply either. Extracts of these cereals have long been considered important by allergists working abroad. As yet they are provided by only two of the firms involved in the British field, one of whom lists four and the other all five. Clinical experience of their importance will take time to accumulate.

Barley (Hordeum secalinum). Cultivated barley is to be found in most areas of England and Wales and specific parts of Scotland. The pollen is encountered in the air during June and July.

Maize (Zea mays). White maize is not grown as frequently as other cereals. It may be found in southern and eastern England and as far north as Yorkshire. Pollination generally occurs in July and August.

Oats (Avena fatua). Cultivated oats are grown throughout the British Isles, although rarely in Wales or Ireland. The pollinating period extends from July to September.

Rye (Secale cereali). Widely cultivated in temperate regions throughout the world, although not grown in the British Isles as frequently as in Europe. Pollinates between June and September. This pollen normally cross-reacts with rye grass (*Lolium perenne*).

Wheat (Triticum sativum). Cultivated fields of wheat are to be found in low-lying areas of Britain and in temperate regions of Europe. Pollination occurs between June and September depending on the local weather conditions.

Weeds

Not all the allergens which affect man are equally noticeable and the non-cultivated plants known as weeds are inevitable intruders even in the best-kept gardens. Certain of these are highly important allergens which are to be considered when grass pollen seems not to be the full answer to a patients summer symptoms or when an extended hay fever season exists. Where an allergy to weeds is suspected but no particular one is indicated the patient may be tested with a weed mix, which one of the firms lists: if this is positive tests may be instigated in order to determine the specific weed causing the allergy.

Dandelion (Taraxacum officinale). Abundant throughout the British Isles and northern hemisphere in pastures, meadows, lawns, waysides and waste places, with pollination occuring from March through till October.

Mugwort (Artemisia vulgaris). Found in waste places, waysides and hedgerows throughout the British Isles, with pollen being produced between July and September.

Nettle (Urtica dioica). The stinging nettle is abundant throughout the British Isles and may be found in temperate regions of the northern hemisphere, particularly where the ground is covered with litter or rubble, but also in hedgerows, woods, grassy places and fens and near buildings. Pollination occurs from June to August, usually showing a biphasic tendency. The pollen grain is large and a lower count than grass pollen will cause symptoms.

Pellitory (Parietaria officinalis). Although widely distributed pellitory-of-the wall tends to be rather local in England, Wales and Ireland, while rare in Scotland. Usually found in cracks in old walls and rocks and hedgebanks, with pollination occuring from June to October.

Plantain (Plantago lanceolata). Found in grassy places on neutral and acid soils, with general distribution throughout the British Isles and Europe. Pollinates from April till August.

Ragweed (Amrbosia artemisiifolia). This weed is uncommon as yet in Britain, but is widely established in America where, particularly on the west coast of the United States, it is the chief cause of hay fever. Many former residents of the United States may mention this pollen when consulting elsewhere. As yet they can be reassured that it has a minimal significance here.

Flowers

Clinical experience suggests that patients who show an allergic response to flowers are often more sensitive to other pollen allergens, particularly grass. However, when an allergy to flowers is suspected, particularly among patients whose hay fever symptoms appear late in the season, a flower mix may be used as the initial test: if it is positive, individual flowers may then be tested.

Flowers which have heavy pollen, such as roses, are unlikely to cause allergies under normal conditions, as the pollen falls to the ground. Similarly insect-pollinated flowers, generally the most colourful ones, have sticky-surfaced pollen grains, which are not generally air-borne, and the same applies. Some other flowers self-pollinate: other plants which have bulbs or corms reproduce vegetatively in part and their pollen is not significant. Many flowers have a perfume, designed to attract insects, and this may itself cause symptoms in patients. However, in the view of the authors such symptoms are generally non-specific hyperactivity, a side-effect engendered by allergy and not truly allergic in themselves.

This list represents the flowers considered by the authors to have some possible clinical significance.

Michaelmas daisy (Aster sp.). To be found in locations extending throughout Britain and Europe with a pollinating period extending from August to September.

Chrysanthemum sp. A cultivated annual with flowers in a variety of colours and pollination occurring from June to August.

Golden rod (Solidago virgaurea). Common in dry woods and grassland and rocks, cliffs and hedgebanks throughout the British Isles, although rare in the south-east. Pollinates from July to September.

Marguerite or daisy (Chrysanthemum leucanthemum). Found commonly on grassland throughout the British Isles, with pollination from June till August.

Wallflower (Cheiranthus sp.). A variety of these flowers are cultivated and some are hybrids (which are often sterile). Those which are not have various pollination forms from April till June and July.

Trees

An allergy to a tree pollen may be suspected when the patient has symptoms similar to hay fever but at the wrong time of the year. Trees pollinate in the United Kingdom between February at the earliest and June at the latest. In some parts of Europe, where grass is less abundant, tree pollens cause the bulk of hay fever symptoms. While the detailed history may reveal that a particular species of tree is causing symptoms, the usual course of action is to use mixes. When a positive result occurs the particular tree may then be identified by using the individual components of the mixture, or in certain cases using extracts of additional trees. Heavy and sticky pollens, such as pine, are unlikely to be inhaled and are, therefore, unlikely to be causative allergens. However, pine trees are associated with a resin called *colophony*. As yet no satisfactory tests exist for this substance, known to be the cause of industrial asthma, but when they are it is probable that we will attach greater importance to it.

Alder (Alnus sp.). Common throughout the British Isles and south Scandinavia and found in waste places, in woods and by lakes and streams up to 500 metres above sea level. Pollinates February to March in Britain and April to May in Scandinavia. The catkins of this tree are well known and, together with hazel, are usually the earliest British pollens.

Ash (Fraxinus sp.). Found on chalky soils in the wetter parts of the British Isles and Scandinavia and in oak woods, scrub and hedges. Pollination occurs from April to May.

Beech (Fagus sylvatica). Although found predominantly in south-east England, it occurs throughout the British Isles, particularly in chalk and limestone soils. Found in south Scandinavia. Pollinates April to May.

Birch (Betula sp.). Found in woods on lighter soils and heathland throughout Britain, although the silver birch predominates in southern England. Pollination occurs from April to May. In Europe it is to be found southwards from Iceland and north Russia. In Scandinavia this tree pollen is the most important allergen of all, exceeding grass pollen in reactivity.

Elder (Sambucus nigra). Common throughout the British Isles and found in woods, scrub, roadsides and waste places. Found in Europe from Scandinavia southwards. Pollinates during June and July.

Elm (Ulmus sp.). Found through England and Europe to 67°N, although less common in the north, and grows in hedges and by roads. Pollinates in February and March in Britain and April and May in Scandinavia. Obviously elm pollen has diminished in recent years due to the ravages of Dutch elm disease. However, it should not be ignored as there are several varieties of elm and in some areas the species is re-establishing itself by regrowth from the roots.

False acacia (Robinia pseudo-acacia). Largely a cultivated tree in Britain, although sometimes planted in thickets. Pollination is in June, overlapping with the grass pollen season.

Hazel (Corylus avellana). Common throughout the British Isles in woods, scrub and hedges. Pollinates from January to April. This is usually the earliest pollen in the United Kingdom and produces the long catkins seen by the roadside in February in southern England.

Hawthorn (Crataegus sp.). Common throughout England, although rare in the north of Scotland. Grows on peaty and acid soils and occurs in scrub and planted extensively in hedgerows. Grows up to 600 metres above sea level. Pollinates in May and June.

Horse chestnut (Aesculus hippocastomum). Found throughout the British Isles, both as a cultivated tree and self sown in deciduous woodland. Pollinates in May to June.

Oak (Quercus sp.). A native tree of Britain found in woods and hedgerows up to 500 metres above sea level, particularly in clay and loam soils. Common in Scandinavia. This tree may reach a great height when well established and the flowers are very small and insignificant, leading one to forget that it can contribute to the pollen problem. Pollinates in April and May in Britain and June in Scandinavia.

Plane or London plane (Platanus orientale). Although not a native of Britain, plane has been planted here, especially in towns, as it stands up better than other varieties to atmospheric pollution. It pollinates during April and May. It is a not insignificant allergen, especially in London in residents or workers in the City.

Poplar (Populus sp.). Various species are to be found in most areas of the British Isles, although it does not grow naturally in damp and wet areas. Pollination occurs from the end of February to early April.

Sycamore (Acer pseudoplatanus). Grows in woods and hedges and plantations throughout the British Isles with pollination occurring from April to June.

Willow (Salix sp.*).* Although a number of different varieties exist, all grow by streams and rivers, marshes and fens and wet woods, although this is now becoming a common garden species. Pollination occurs from April to May.

Moulds or fungi

The range of moulds that occur naturally in the United Kingdom is very wide and varied, but the following are those which, clinically speaking, seem to be responsible for the majority of mould allergies. Where the case history does not include a specific mould, fungi mixes may, or in the case of perennial allergies should, be used in the diagnosis; individual moulds may be tested if a positive reaction occurs. Other moulds may be suggested by the case history and may be tested for on an individual basis.

Moulds have a considerable importance to the allergist, but are not well known to the general public and lack common English names. Often, therefore, patients will require explanations of why they are to be tested for them. They often cause symptoms when no pollen is in the air.

Alternaria tenuis. Found on a variety of cultivated plants including wheat and as early blight on potatoes, with sporulation (the equivalent to a mould of pollination) occurring in warm dry weather with a peak in August or September. *Alternaria* is the fungus most commonly encountered in patients with seasonal rhinitis or asthma.

Aspergillus sp. Plant débris such as compost heaps and stacks of hay and straw produce large numbers of spores which may be liberated producing a high local level. A high incidence occurs during the winter months, possibly due to widespread distribution of decaying leaves. *Aspergillus* also occurs as a black mould on cotton bolls, fruits and vegetables. May be found in damp old houses. *Aspergillus fumigatus* is a mould frequently associated with type III reaction: where a positive prick test to this substance is elicited, this possibility should always be borne in mind. A non-immediate reaction to *Aspergillus fumigatus* requires an evaluation by an allergist of considerable expertise.

Botrytis. Occurs as the common grey mould on a variety of vegetables: potatoes, cucumbers and particularly strawberries. Some people who think they are allergic to strawberries may, in fact, suffer from a *Botrytis* sensitivity. The fungus thrives in a damp, cool, atmosphere and occurs outdoors mainly in the autumn.

Candida albicans. A white mould which occurs as a food yeast and causes diseases like thrush and occasionally athlete's foot. Grows best in a warm, wet environment.

Chaetomium. To be found on straw, wet paper, cotton fibres and dung and likely to be encountered at any time of year.

Cladosporium herbarum. Occurs widely with sporulation in the hay fever season and the summer, causing mainly asthma and to a lesser extent, nasal symptoms in the majority of patients sensitive to this fungus. Peak annual concentration of the spores occurs during July and August. This mould often contributes to hay fever, especially in those who do not seem to have symptoms which coincide with the grass pollen count.

Curvularia. Although not found as frequently as the other moulds, this may occur as spots on corn and other cereals from June to September.

Fusarium. A white or colourless fungus which is commonly found in a wide variety of environments. May be found as the dry rot on potatoes, 'cabbage yellow', tomato wilt, cereal foot rot, cotton wilt and Panama disease of bananas. The occurrence tends, therefore, to be local rather than generalized.

Helminthosporium. Occurs as a parasitic fungus on many cereals, particularly wheat and barley. May also occur on decomposing plant matter. Spores are air-borne, mainly during August and September.

Merulius. See *Serpula.*

Micropolyspora faeni. Occurs in piles of damp hay which are undisturbed causing the mouldy appearance and produces heat and decomposition. May sporulate at any time of year and more typically in late autumn and winter. Responsible largely for the condition known as farmers' lung.

Mucor. Found frequently on stored food, this mould thrives on damp substances and may also be found as a constituent of house dust, especially in older homes.

Neurospora. Normally encountered in bakeries and known as bakery mould or red bread mould. Also widely used in genetic and physiological research laboratories.

Penicillium. As the name implies, this is the mould from which penicillin was originally discovered. Some strains are still used for the production of this antibiotic. It is commonly found as the blue and green moulds of apples and citrus fruits and may occur in house dust. Spores are present in the air at most times of the year.

Phoma. Occurs on beet as 'black leg' and on citrus fruits as 'black spot'. It is also found on the stems of lavender, marigolds and other summer flowers, and on decomposing nettles.

Pullularia. Sporulating in the summer, this mould is found on vegetables and fruit and damp painted surfaces.

Rhizopus. A common parasite of mature fruits and vegetables; it may also occur on stale bread and other surfaces.

Serpula lacrimans. This mould does have a well known lay name as it is the cause of dry rot. This occurs in the woodwork of buildings especially where there is both moisture and a lack of ventilation. Dry rot is commonly associated with the older buildings but may occur in quite new houses where the above conditions prevail. This mould attacks the house; the spore attacks the patient causing asthma and rhinitis.

Sporobolomyces. This fungus is sometimes present in wines and wine products and may be implicated in apparent allergy to alcohol. It also occurs outdoors, sporulating in warm damp conditions especially at dew fall and during and just after light summer rain. It is associated mainly with allergic rhinitis and often affects patients in damp places such as near trees, rivers or lakes and when camping.

Trichophyton. A parasitic fungus and the cause of tinea pedis in man.

Ustilago. Commonly occurs as the 'smut' on cereals, especially wheat, causing a dark powdery deposit on the grain. May also occur on oats, maize and grasses. Sporulation is maximal in late summer.

Other Inhalants

House dust. For at least a century allergic responses to dust have been known. However, we must consider exactly what we mean by dust: it is the particulate debris which accumulates in any given area and as such will inevitably reflect the materials in the environment of the dust, and only those materials. This, of course, implies correctly that dust from different places will be different. Thus, dust from an engineering factory may show concrete fragments, rust particles and metal dust. In an office the dust will show paper fragments. The dust with which we are mainly concerned is household dust. This contains fabric fragments from furnishings, mould spores, and shed skin from humans and pets and many patients may be sensitized to this mixture. However, the most important constituent of house dust is the microscopic mite called the house dust mite; generally treatment of house dust allergy on its own is now contemplated only in circumstances where the patient does not react positively to the house dust mite.

House dust mite (Dermatophagoides pteronyssinus). This creature has been known to science for a very long time. However, its significance was not appreciated until 1964 and reliable extracts for skin testing were not available until 1974, although extracts of *Dermatophagoides farinae* (grown on flour) were available before this. This microscopic transparent mite lives exclusively on a diet of human skin scale and abounds, therefore, wherever man sheds scales. This mainly means in the bedroom and around the mattress, but favorite armchairs and carpets where children play can also be places where the mite occurs. Cars and lorry cabs with nylon cloth upholstery will also trap mites. What these places have in common is a retentive surface and the presence of man for a long enough period to shed a significant number of scales. The mite prefers coldish, damp houses and is averse to bright sunlight. The peak breeding season is in middle to late summer, but dead mites, which cause the same problem as living ones, are maximal in the late summer and early autumn. One should note that there are several other species of mite in house dust, some of which may later assume an increased importance. At present it is felt that *Dermatophagoides pteronyssinus* is the most significant.

Hay dust. This is found in stables or where livestock are housed. This includes pet rabbits and guinea-pigs. The dust may be brought home on clothing by agricultural workers or by children riding horses and ponies.

Wheat flour is used very widely both in bakeries and in the home. However, it is important to note that as an inhalant it can cause rhinitis and asthma, sometimes of considerable severity.

Animals. Since time immemorial man has lived in close association with animals; even today in an industrial society the range of contacts can be truly amazing if a detailed enquiry is made. Pets at home and at school and products made from animal materials must all be sought.

Feathers. May be found more frequently in the home than on birds, as fillings in pillows, cushions, duvets and quilts and in upholstery. Most such feathers are mixed and common species involved are chicken, duck and goose. However, feathers are also used as dusters, because their design makes them very good at trapping dust, and the majority of patients who give a positive response to feathers will give a better one to house dust and an even better one to the house dust mite. It should not be forgotten that the mite was first isolated from dust from an old feather pillow.

Cage birds. A few years ago this meant mainly budgerigars, canaries and the occasional parrot. Now an increasing number of exotic birds may be found in the home, including parrots, parakeets, zebra and other tropical finches, Java sparrows and many others. Commercially only budgerigar extract is available. Allergy to cage birds is not simply due to feathers. The droppings which dry off and are blown as dust throughout the home can cause rhinitis and severe asthma, marked by late reaction. Where such reactions are suspected, the services of an expert allergist are required.

Pigeons. Commonly kept in lofts rather than in homes, pigeons present problems identical to cage birds particularly in the north of England.

Cat. Allergy to the domestic cat is one of the best known animal allergies and these animals can cause the whole range of allergic responses (see Chapter 2). It is probable that more than one allergen is involved and saliva, skin scales and fur are implicated.

Dog. This animal is responsible for engendering a similar range of allergic responses, although in many cases responsiveness is less than for the cat. However, when an individual patient is allergic to a dog the reaction can be just as severe as in cat allergy.

With both cat and dog some, but not all, patients show a response to some members of the species but are apparently tolerant to others. The authors feel that there should be an awareness that such responsiveness exists, although its nature and significance are not known.

Hamsters, guinea-pigs and gerbils. These small rodents are very commonly kept as domestic pets by children and are frequently found in infant and junior schools. They are also found in research laboratories. All may give rise to quite severe allergic reactions which, in the case of animal handlers in laboratories, may be such as to warrant a change of occupation. There is no commercial extract available for gerbil at the time of writing. These creatures are frequently bedded on straw or hay which may also give rise to allergic responses; occasional patients may be found to be allergic to this material and not to their pet.

Horse. The horse is an animal capable of engendering a severe degree of allergic response, not infrequently coupled with an adamant refusal on the behalf of its besotted female teenage sufferer to take any reasonable steps with regard to the allergen. The problem may, however, extend from one member of the family who rides horses to cause illness in other members of the family from dander and hair brought home on clothing. The house may contain horse hair in mattresses, upholstery, especially in older furniture, and even plaster in old houses. Horse serum is present in a number of vaccines in very small amounts and some degree of rather unreliable cross-reactivity does occur with horse dander prick extracts.

Rabbits. These are usually outdoor pets and much the same comments apply to them as to guinea-pigs, although the degree of reactivity is usually less. However, the pelts are found as fur coats and in wool, especially fur from the angora rabbit which is used in manufacturing fashion clothing. Rabbit paws are occasionally turned into rather macabre jewellery items.

Sheep wool. This is encountered by most patients largely as clothing and furnishings, including floor coverings. However, the unprocessed wool is more allergenic than the finished article and worse reactions may be engendered by sheep-skin rugs and coats and obviously by the farming industry. Dyed wool may cause problems because of dye allergy as well as wool sensitivity. Some patients may be only dye-sensitive.

Cow. Allergic responses to leather as a contact substance are common, frequently due to processing. However, fur and abattoir workers may become sensitized to cow epithelia.

Animal parasites. Human allergy to animal fleas, ticks and mites may occur, although as yet no extract for any of these substances is available in the United Kingdom. One such deserves special mention as it is at present as unknown to the medical and nursing professions as it is common knowledge to every veterinary general practitioner and his nurse. This is *Chelytiella*, sometimes known as the rabbit fur mite. This is a poor name, as it is by no means confined to rabbits but occurs in cats, dogs and other small animals, especially kittens and puppies. It is more common in spring and autumn. The mite used to be considered a commensal but is now thought to promote skin conditions in the animal host. It has also been incriminated in man as a cause of urticaria and eczema and may well be much more important than we once thought.

Stinging insects. In Great Britain the chief problems are caused by bees and wasps, although from time to time horseflies and hornets may be involved, as may the bites of mosquitoes. In all subjects a local reaction to the sting will take place; the material injected is a venom, the procedure being intended as a defence mechanism for the insect. The local reaction does not constitute an allergy. Some subjects, however, become sensitized to the venom and develop generalized symptoms of rash, oedema or anaphylaxis which may be severe and can cause loss of life. The oedema can affect the larynx and this is always a life-threatening emergency.

Skin testing for insect allergy may itself be accompanied by an anaphylactic reaction. Many allergists of experience will omit this step, therefore, if a clear history has been obtained which is regarded as sufficient to identify the insect concerned. Because of the risks attending such testing, the investigation of insect allergy should remain in the hands of experienced allergists working in units where good resuscitation facilities are at hand.

Foods

Allergy to foods is becoming increasingly well known, and may coexist in patients with other allergic problems. Some of the problems which are clinically associated with foods have been covered in Chapter 2. Almost any food can be involved, as may food additives, such as preservatives and dyes. Prick and intradermal tests for foods have long been available but controversy rages about whether these are of value. In the authors' opinion they are not. Laboratory tests are also available for some, but not all, foods. As yet these are not either freely available or of undoubted reliability.

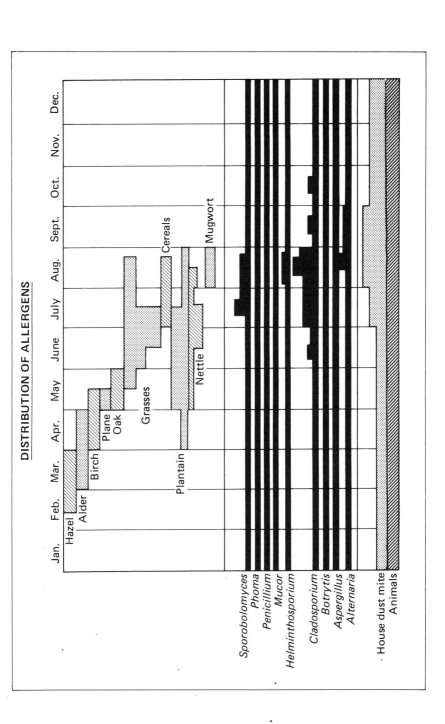

DISTRIBUTION OF ALLERGENS

DISTRIBUTION CHART

The authors feel that many workers in the field of allergy will find use for a monthly chart which shows the approximate distribution of allergens as they occur through the year. The chart is, of necessity, approximate; for seasonal allergens year-by-year variation occurs and the season in the south of England is not identical to that in the north of Scotland. However, it will form a general guide and is based on the pollen and mould experiences of southern England, the area local to the authors.

5

The Case History

The taking of the case history is probably the most important factor in the successful diagnosis of allergy. Much time, effort and expense can be saved if the history is taken carefully and in depth. Having said this, it becomes obvious that it is not a diagnostic step which should be hurried and it is essential to make sure that sufficient time is allowed to provide for this when booking clinics.

The patients' first contact with the doctor or nurse in the clinic is very often when the history is taken and it is important to make sure that they are relaxed and not over-anxious, otherwise they will often forget points which are important or else take a long time remembering the timing of certain symptoms. The answers to your questions are not always straightforward. For example, patients with perennial allergies and hay fever may present a confused history which leads the allergist or nurse to assume that either the perennial or the seasonal component is the whole complaint.

It may be advisable, in patients with an apparently disconnected history, to keep a symptom chart over a period of several months. This will help to clarify the situation and decide not only the likely substances to which the patient is allergic but also the severity of the reactions. In a busy hospital clinic, however desirable it might be to send the patient away to fill in a chart in this way before attempting to take diagnosis any further, it is not always feasible, as many clinics have a waiting list for appointments of several months. However, in general practice such a procedure is straightforward and easily accepted. Most general practitioners cannot give half an hour at a time to one patient but short consultations between the doctor, nurse and patient soon remedy this.

Several case history charts are produced by the firms manufacturing allergy solutions, notably Bencard, Dome Laboratories and E. Merck. Some clinics produce their own charts. The charts are a very useful guide to the taking of a history and mapping out of skin tests. A history chart devised by one of the authors is reproduced here for guidance.

Using the chart as a guide, take the questions one at a time, remembering the various factors which can be important such as housing, occupation and the forms in which the reactions present. These have previously been described in Chapter 2.

It should always be borne in mind that the allergy may be a reaction to something of which the patient is particularly fond. The classic example of this is the family pet; when a child is concerned, the presence of a parent during history-taking is essential if an accurate account is to be obtained. However, the parents may find it equally hard to accept that their own interests or hobbies may adversely affect their child. Similarly a person's occupation may cause problems which might necessitate changing a job from which immense satisfaction or financial rewards are derived. Thus the doctor or nurse, when taking a history, must be aware of the possibility of concealment of facts.

Some nurses will be required to decide on the basis of the history which skin tests are indicated. They will find an account of characteristics of individual allergens and pollen charts a great advantage in completing this task. Such an account is given in Chapter 4.

It is the authors' firm opinion that no nurse should be expected to take case histories without previous instruction. This can be in the form of observing and then being observed by a doctor or nurse well versed in the art. In the absence of such skills, a very great expenditure of time will clearly be required in learning safe history-taking and in this learning time mistakes will be made. Fortunately most allergy departments are always willing to provide such assistance to doctors and nurses.

In addition there are moves afoot at the time of writing to make available recognized courses of instruction in allergy for nursing staff. Some commercial firms do provide courses and their representatives will pass on queries to the appropriate departments.

ALLERGY CASE HISTORY

DATE .... TAKEN BY ....

SURNAME .... Hospital No.
(Block Letters)
FORENAMES

Address
Ward/Hosp
Sex M.   F.
     M. S. W.

Hay Fever ☐   Non-seasonal Asthma ☐

Seasonal Asthma ☐   Other ☐

Perennial Rhinitis ☐   Sneezing ☐

Discharge ☐   Blockage ☐

PLEASE RING APPROPRIATE ITEMS

Severity of symptoms

   MILD   MODERATE   SEVERE

Age at onset ....

Are symptoms – ALL YEAR ROUND   SEASONAL

Are symptoms:

Jan	Feb	Mar	Apr	May	June	July	Aug	Sept	Oct	Nov	Dec

PERENNIAL   SEASONAL

Constant   Intermittent   Immediately on contact   Some hours later

Affected by: WET   DRY   HOT   Both

COLD SUMMER WINTER INDOORS   If seasonal: BETTER IN WET WEATHER Yes/No

OUTDOORS   BETTER INDOORS   Yes/No

                                    Near: TREES GRASS CEREALS WEEDS (Type)

HOME ENVIRONMENT: AGE OF HOUSE..........IN TOWN/COUNTRY   DAMP/DRY

HEAVY FURNISHINGS IN BEDROOM Yes/No   FEATHER PILLOWS/DUVET/EIDERDOWN Yes/No

HORSE HAIR MATTRESS Yes/No

HEATING: Central – Radiators Yes/No   Ducted Warm Air Yes/No

Paraffin/Butane Heaters Yes/No

Other – give details ....

....

<u>WORK ENVIRONMENT</u> JOB...

Affected at work   Yes/No   Materials at work...

<u>ANIMAL CONTACTS</u>   CAT / DOG / GERBIL / HAMSTER etc. / BUDGIES & CAGE BIRDS /

RABBIT / HORSE / COW / SHEEP / POULTRY / OTHER (details)

....

....

<u>FOOD ALLERGIES</u> (Specify) ....

....

....

<u>TYPE OF REACTION</u> ....

....

<u>PAST ALLERGIC HISTORY</u>..

....

<u>FAMILY HISTORY</u> ....

....

PROBLEMS IDENTIFIED

ACTION / TREATMENT

EVALUATION

6

Skin Testing

We now move to skin testing, the step with which the allergist is most commonly associated, both by the lay public and by our non-allergist colleagues, but it is important to realize that this step cannot be taken without adequate knowledge of the previous steps. We must understand our subject and have determined the probable allergens from the patient's history. The authors, as students, were taught that diagnosis comprised three steps: first history, second examination and third, but only third, confirmatory tests.

Skin testing, although a form of examination, is in essence more akin to the third of these steps and as such should confirm the diagnosis made on history rather than be inaugurated by an allergist whose mind remains blank until the results are read.

The term skin testing covers three modes of testing, *prick testing, intradermal testing* and *patch testing*. The solutions employed use a measured amount of allergen dissolved in glycerinated normal saline, with phenol added.

Some comment should be made on the technique of glycerination of skin test solutions. The diluent used in standard inhalant practice is normal saline. Whilst this is obviously a safe substance to introduce into the body, and can easily be sterilized, it offers no resistance to bacterial or viral contamination of the solution and for this reason a small amount of antiseptic material, usually phenol, is added. Although this protects the solution against contamination, it does nothing to preserve the allergen added to the saline, which is likely to change in chemical nature over a period of time. It is to assist in stabilizing the allergen that glycerin is added, usually in a strength of 50%.

PRICK TESTING

Prick testing is the mode currently considered to be the most valuable in the diagnosis of inhalent allergies. There are various ways in which the technique can be carried out and the use of these various techniques will give rise to varying results. In certain parts of the world multiple puncture techniques, or linear scratches, are still carried out, but in the United Kingdom the standard technique is known as the modified prick test. In the authors' view (a view shared by the majority of British allergists), it is essential that a standard technique should be used so as to reduce to a minimum the variation between clinics, caused by varying test techniques.

The modified prick test is carried out as follows. The most suitable site is the flexor side of the forearm. The skin is marked with a ballpoint pen, felt tip pen or skin marker so as to identify and locate the site of each test. A single drop of each test solution is placed adjacent to the marker. It is desirable that this should be dropped rather than dabbed on to the arm to minimize transfer of any contaminants from one patient to the next. Tests should be at least 3 cm apart. A sterile lancet is used for the test, rather than a needle, as the latter is hollow and cannot be wiped clean. If a needle is used, a new one is required for each test, which is an unnecessary expense. Sterile lancets are cheaply available from firms manufacturing allergy test solutions. The lancet is then placed at an acute angle to the skin and a shallow lift is made. The lancet is raised for a second before the skin is released. This is repeated for each drop of solution, the lancet being carefully wiped on dry cotton wool or a paper tissue medical wipe between tests. After the procedure has been completed any excess solution remaining on the skin is removed by blotting the arm with a paper tissue.

The tests are then allowed to incubate. The time interval varies between clinics from a minimum of ten minutes to a maximum of twenty. Some allergists prefer that the arm be exposed during this interval, others that it be covered. The authors prefer the latter and read results after ten minutes. It is felt by us that the warmth and covering reduce the effects of cold and nervousness in inhibiting responsiveness.

The results are then read. Here again wide local variation

TECHNIQUE OF PRICK TESTING

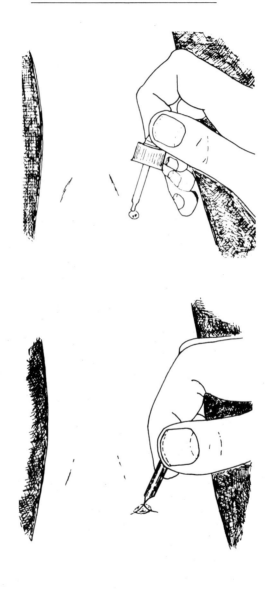

exists in methods of recording what one sees and it is desirable to minimize these. The reaction appears as a white raised weal surrounded by a red flare. At the present time it is the weal that is measured. Most allergists fall back on the rather subjective system of grading weals by a number of plusses; when this is done + or +++ may well mean different things on different days, even in the same clinic. However, an individual operator can become quite consistent with this technique. The weakness is the total lack of comparability between clinics. The advantage is speed in recording results. Some persons use rulers or circular discs to measure the results in millimetres. The disadvantage of this system is that many weals are markedly assymetical. If measurement is to be used the best technique for such responses is to use a millimetre square grid. This is extremely tedious and not really feasible in a busy clinic, although possible for research purposes. The third technique is the adhesive tape transfer method. The weal is delineated by drawing round it exactly with a ballpoint pen. Obviously an error in this drawing will cause mismeasurement. The necessity for exactitude in carrying out this step cannot be stressed too highly. A length of transparent adhesive tape is then pressed down onto the skin lightly but firmly. When this is removed the ink mark will have transferred itself to the tape sufficiently to enable an indelible transfer to be retained; the tape is then stuck down to the case record. By this technique, correctly done, the case records contain exactly what the allergist saw at the time the test was done and exact measurement of this may be carried out at any time in the future that it may be required. Such measurements may be made by any future worker without reference to the original tester.

The authors currently use the +++ technique in practical clinic work because of speed. It is, however, our practice that whenever working together we jointly score the plusses and find thereby that some consistency is obtained. We are, however, considering going on to the tape transfer method for future work and already use this whenever it is felt important to record the results with exactitude.

Having spent some time on the question of exact measurement, it must also be said clearly that prick testing is qualitative rather than quantitive. By this we mean that the presence of a positive test indicates reactivity, but the size is not necessarily as relevant. A 9 mm diameter weal does not necessarily indicate twice as much responsiveness as a 4 mm weal. The skin tests indicate 'atopic status', a commonly used term to describe the possessor of positive skin tests. Such a person may not always have allergic symptoms. Families of allergic patients may have atopic status and positive skin tests without necessarily having hay fever, for example, although they may show a positive skin test to grass pollen. This factor is of extreme importance when it comes to considering treatment and will be discussed further in Chapter 10.

INTRADERMAL TESTING

The next mode of testing to be considered is intradermal testing. For this technique the solutions are dispensed in multi-dose vials, rather than dropper bottles, as they must remain sterile. Only one of the three firms in the British allergy field, Bencard, markets a range of intradermal solutions and their range is less than in former days. This is because the technique is not used in Great Britain as a routine method, but is reserved for certain cases when it is felt that prick testing is not satisfactory. Intradermal testing involves the injection of much larger doses of allergen and in a highly sensitized patient there will be a greater risk of an anaphylactic reaction. Furthermore, because of the volume of material injected there is a greater risk of a false-positive result. For both these reasons intradermal solutions are usually marketed at a lower strength than prick solutions. In certain Continental countries the technique is still used as the basic method. In Great Britain research is revealing certain conditions where intradermal testing may be indicated and the technique may then be re-established; if so the precise amounts required on injection will be made clear by those advocating the revised procedure.

PATCH TESTING

This is a quite different technique, one which has no place in the diagnosis of inhalant allergies, but is usually essential in the diagnosis of atopic eczema and contact dermatitis. It is occasionally of use in urticaria. Usually in these conditions prick testing yields little information of value.

As with prick testing a measured amount of the contact is dissolved in a suitable base which is usually greasy. Petroleum jelly is standard. The tests employed are in some ways more standardized than those used in prick testing as a European standard battery is usually used. This may be augmented by supplementary tests. Several firms manufacture test material. Unfortunately to get a complete set it is often necessary to patronise more than one such firm. However, in some cases they advise an equivalent and since dispensing some of these is easier than preparing prick test extracts many hospital pharmacists make test material for their own allergy clinics.

The tests are usually applied to the back, as quite a number are involved. As one of the substances to which tests are being carried out is the base material used in adhesive strapping it is necessary to apply the test strips using Sellotape or Micropore strapping which is unlikely to promote a reaction in itself. The tests are applied using a small quantity of ointment which is then covered for a measured period during which it is left in close contact with the skin. A suitable method of applying the battery can be devised for oneself, but commercial firms do make excellent prepared test stips, which can usually be supplied by those who sell the test battery, and most clinics prefer to use them.

Variation enters the procedure in the length of time for which the test is applied. Some clinicians apply the patches for 24 hours and then read after three days, repeating the procedure for a further two days. Many others leave the test application for three days and then read the results.

From the patient's viewpoint the most important thing is keeping the tests on for the requisite period. We include in this chapter a set of instructions to patients which are clear and have been sucessfully used in the Reading Hospitals for some years past. They need, of course, to be supplemented by detailed explanation to the patient.

Interpretation of the results requires extreme expertise, as there are irritant results and false-positives to contend with.

INSTRUCTIONS TO PATIENTS WHO HAVE BEEN PATCH TESTED

To establish whether you are allergic to certain materials or substances, a series of patch tests have been applied to the skin of your back. These patch tests might identify the cause of an allergic eczema.

The patch tests must be left in place for two days and two nights.

Do not take a bath or shower, nor wash your back whilst the patch tests are in position.

Avoid excessive exercise which causes heavy perspiration.

Avoid friction or rubbing of the patch tests which may loosen them.

Do not expose the test area to the sun.

Should the patch tests become loose, please replace them with sticky tape in the original position and inform the doctor or nurse at your next visit that you have had to restick the tapes.

The clinician is looking for a true eczema reaction to establish a positive.

Clearly, therefore, any nurse carrying out patch testing will need to have had practical in job training by an experienced and competent authority.

In the authors' view the same applies to prick testing. Although the techniques can be described in a book, at least one practical demonstration is desirable before commencing work. As we have said before, most allergy clinics provide this service.

7

Laboratory Tests

In addition to history-taking and skin testing it is now possible to undertake further procedures to confirm a diagnosis of allergy. Such confirmation will not always be necessary: a clear-cut case of hay fever, for example, will not need laboratory investigation. However, it may be essential, for example, for a perennial conjunctivitis where no clear-cut allergic diagnosis emerges.

EOSINOPHIL COUNT

The simplest procedure, and one for which all laboratories are equipped, is to test for eosinophils. We have seen in Chapter 3 the essential place of these in the chain of events taking place in allergy. They can be stained with the dye eosin and are then easily recognized in blood and secretions under the microscope. A differential white blood count will occasionally reflect the patient's allergic status by having an increased eosinophil count. The usual level is 3–5% of the total. However, an increased count in not infallible evidence of allergy as there are other cases of increased blood eosinophilia. Far more convincing is to measure the level in potentially allergic secretions. For practical purposes these are sputum, nasal washings and ophthalmic secretions. In non-allergic conditions these contain mainly neutrophils and occasional polymorphs. In allergy there may be a rich secretion of eosinophils of such a degree as to establish without doubt the allergic nature of the exudate. This investigation is cheap, easily collected and processed in any laboratory. It is, however, non-specific: whilst it points to an allergic diagnosis it provides no clue as to the individual allergen.

IMMUNE STATUS

Additional information may be gathered by examining the patient's immune status by a direct measurement of his antibodies (immunoglobulins). As we have seen in Chapter 3 information about the large molecule IgG, IgA and IgM has been available for many years and some information may be gained by a measurement of these factors. This again should be available as a routine investigation in most hospital laboratories. Measurement of these values will indicate the presence of immunodeficiency or of infection and may point to its nature as being viral or bacterial.

A rise in IgG as measured by this means is not a measurement of the efficacy of allergy treatment or blocking antibodies as such responses need a more exact estimation of IgG subclasses which is not feasible in the normal laboratory service.

The most useful information, however, will come from a measurement of IgE. This can be achieved in a number of ways. The most feasible measurement in a peripheral hospital is a *total IgE*. Such a measurement will include IgE from sources other than allergic, but it does give useful guidance in the majority of cases. Not all hospitals are yet equipped to do this, but if not they may well be able to refer specimens on to a nearby unit which can. The test itself can be done by two different techniques; the RIST (radio-immunosorbant test) is probably more accurate for our purposes. However, the alternative technique, immunofluorescence, may be made available more economically. It is essential to recognize that results from the two methods cannot be compared with each other. The result has a useful if limited predictive value and the authors use it in cases where the result on prick testing does not illuminate the diagnosis. A level of 10 IU, or below, coupled with negative skin tests is used to exclude allergy, as a level of this order will only, with extreme rarity, be associated with an allergic diagnosis. By contrast a level above 100 IU indicates a probably allergic diagnosis until proved otherwise. The techniques subsequently used will be detailed in Chapter 8.

A measurement of total IgE is thus available, but far more helpful, where possible, is the measurement of *specific IgE*. In

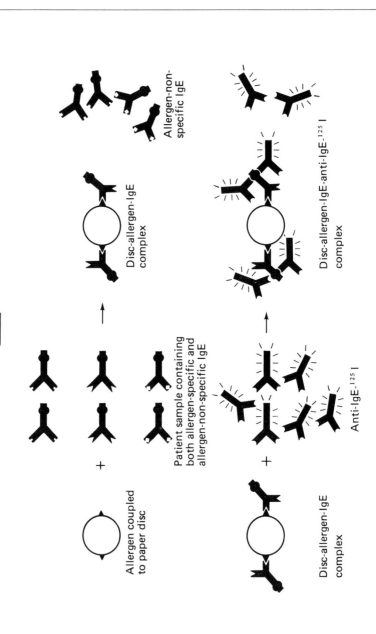

RAST

PRIST

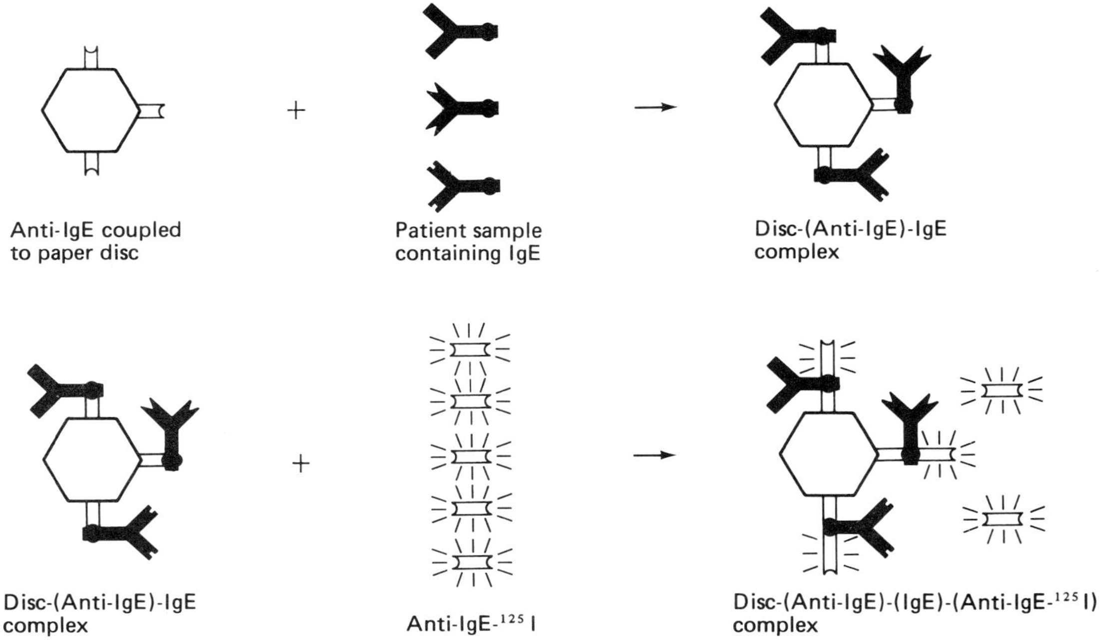

Anti-IgE coupled to paper disc

+

Patient sample containing IgE

→

Disc-(Anti-IgE)-IgE complex

Disc-(Anti-IgE)-IgE complex

+

Anti-IgE-^{125}I

→

Disc-(Anti-IgE)-(IgE)-(Anti-IgE-^{125}I) complex

this technique the level of IgE specific to, say, grass pollen or house dust mite is measured directly. Here we know not only that the IgE is allergic, but also the allergen that is involved. The test involved is known as RAST (radio-allergo-sorbant test); as its name implies, like RIST, it is a method that involves the use of radio-isotopes. For those interested the processes involved in both RIST and RAST are detailed on pp. 58 and 59. Some centres have contemplated the use of RAST as an alternative to skin testing; indeed, if cost is no object (it is a very expensive test, using both expensive equipment and highly skilled technicians), this may in the future be a sound policy. At present, however, only a somewhat limited range of antigens is commercially available and the procedure works better for some than others. Thus the authors conclude that at present it is a useful adjunct, especially at a research level, rather than a complete replacement of existing skin testing methods. By contrast, the results of immunological are often found to be useful in food allergies, where skin testing is unreliable.

PRECIPITINS

The final laboratory parameter widely used is the measurement of precipitins. Chapter 3 states that precipitating antibodies are associated with type III responses and that this phenomenon is commonest in bronchopulmonary aspergillosis. Where a skin test is positive, and preferably where evidence of a non-immediate response also present, estimations of precipitins may be requested. These have been found, experimentally, not only in aspergillosis and farmers' lung, but in association with a wide variety of mould problems such as mushroom-workers' lung and malt-workers' lung, and also with allergens such as house dust mite and even grass pollen. The evaluation of such tests requires skill and they are available only at certain reference laboratories. They may serve as confirmatory evidence of a notifiable and compensatable industrial disease, but a firm diagnosis requires a clinician whose opinion is established enough to withstand evaluation by an industrial medical tribunal.

In time, we have no doubt, immunology will require the use of further tests. The authors feel, however, that until allergy is better established the availability of even these tests may take some time to develop and that these tests are all that need be described as yet in a chapter such as this.

8

Further Tests

We have now considered the usual steps which are undertaken to establish a diagnosis of allergy and the laboratory tests which can help to substantiate that diagnosis: we have also seen some of the limitations of these steps. Accurate history is always, of course, incontrovertible, as it comprises the statement by the patient of the real problem as it affects him or her. Subsequently one attempts to confirm this by skin testing, although in some instances there is no precise extract available to confirm the diagnosis. Equally it is possible that the patient may be a non-skin-reactor and that skin tests may, therefore, be completely unhelpful.

Consequently we have reviewed in Chapter 7 the further steps that may be undertaken to establish a diagnosis of allergy: you will remember that many of these are non-specific and do not indicate any individual antigen and that those which are specific are not freely available in most centres.

Thus there are occasions when the allergist will require further tests in order to obtain a clear-cut answer. You will note that the phrase used is 'the allergist'. These tests generally carry increased risks to the patient. Whilst there is an undoubted place for the nurse or technician in such procedures, it is a more circumscribed role and they all need rigorous medical super-vision. The reason for this added caution is not hard to see. In previous modes of testing, with the exception of patch testing, we have been carrying out an indirect test. Here, however, we are seeking to reproduce directly the disease from which the patient suffers by stimulus with the allergen to which it is suspected he or she may be sensitized. In skin testing, the risk of anaphylaxis, whilst present, is minimal. In nasal and bronchial challenge, in particular, it is far from minimal and should constantly be in the forefront of the minds of all allergy workers during the test interval.

CONJUNCTIVAL CHALLENGE

The first of these further tests we shall consider is conjunctival challenge. Here a drop or drops (usually one only) are instilled into the conjunctival sac. If the patient is capable of producing an ophthalmic reaction to the allergen it will be manifest within the same interval as a prick skin test: a positive result in such circumstances is much nearer to the symptoms of the patient than a prick test is in hay fever and because of its direct simplicity you may wonder why it is but rarely used. There are a number of reasons. Firstly only sterile drops should be used in the eye and our prick test extracts, unless freshly opened for this test, cannot be regarded as sterile. Secondly, we have seen that upon occasion they eye can exhibit reactions of great severity which can even result in loss of vision. It is clearly undesirable to risk this unless there is a good justification for the test. Thirdly, it is possible, as we have seen, to perform a large battery of skin tests in one session, whereas a conjunctival challenge can only be performed for a single allergen at one consultation. It is obviously necessary to leave an untreated eye to act as a control. Some allergists prefer to use a control solution before embarking on tests, but it is probably unwise to use glycerinated drops in the ophthalmic tests and it seems to the authors unnecessary to challenge the eye with a drop of normal saline. However, it has always seemed to the authors that the results obtained by this means can be obtained more satisfactorily by other means and this procedure is not in use in our clinics.

NASAL CHALLENGE

When a further direct test is required it is to nasal challenge that we turn. The principle is obviously the same, in that a measured dose of allergen is introduced into the nose and the result is measured after ten to twenty minutes. The procedure is fraught with the same risk of anaphylaxis and again carries the disadvantage that only a limited number of tests can be carried out at one consultation. Some authorities use both nares, which clearly speeds diagnosis if a number of allergens are to be tried, but has the disadvantage of removing the untreated side comparison. It has been suggested that glycerinated solutions may be sensitizers and it is thus felt wise to limit to a moderate number the total nasal challenges to be carried out. Work has been carried out in a number of centres showing that repeated nasal challenges can produce a measure of hyposensitization and thus it is essential that a nasal challenge be done correctly as it cannot necessarily be repeated for that allergen with the same validity.

A wide variety of techniques have been used for this test and an individual allergist who carries out the procedure will have such a protocol, together with good reasons for carrying out the method selected. It is thus not appropriate to describe any individual method, since in the authors' view this procedure is not one that should in any way be initiated by a nurse or technician. However, a final point that may be made is with regard to the strength of test solutions. Some authorities use diluted skin test extract and these will therefore require clear labelling and storage so that they cannot be confused with prick extracts. In such cases there is a good case to be made for the doctor and nurse or technician jointly checking the material before it is introduced into the patient.

So far we have discussed techniques which, although requiring greater expertise and carrying greater risks than prick testing, can nevertheless be carried out on out-patients. The next two methods, in the authors' view, should be practiced only on patients in a hospital in-patient bed where practised resident medical staff are on site for the whole 24 hours. There are two reasons for this, the first being the risks to the patient, and the second being that the value of the test is directly proportional to the accuracy of observation that follows and it is our clear duty to ensure that a high risk test need only be carried out once. If a patient reports a consequence which has not been observed because of lack of skilled medical cover the procedure may have to be repeated. *This should never be necessary.*

BRONCHIAL CHALLENGE

Bronchial challenge is, in essence, a similar procedure to nasal conjunctival challenge, in that potentially allergenic material is directly exposed to the test side and the consequences monitored. Conventionally it is usual to observe such patients for at least 48 hours after challenge, as non-immediate reactions are commonly seen. The illustration on p. 68 shows such a response as measured by peak flow readings sequentially obtained. In the authors' view such long-term monitoring is equally desirable in nasal challenge, as similar phenomena in terms of allergic activity do occur and will be recorded only if sought. However, the immediate importance of a nasal reaction is clearly less than the hazard of producing experimental asthma, as the patient may require medical treatment if the condition progresses to cause some respiratory embarrassment.

Nevertheless, although there are very considerable risks in bronchial challenge tests it must be realized that the procedure elicits information which cannot be obtained by any other means and in skilled hands it is an essential tool, particularly for the investigation of non-immediate responses and especially type III responses. These, as we have seen in Chapter 3, are tissue-damaging and provide an additional reason for ensuring that such a test need only be carried out on a single occasion.

In such a test the nurse or technician will be required to work as part of a well informed and extremely disciplined team. It is, therefore, essential to find out in advance exactly what is required of a team member.

OCCUPATIONAL TESTING

Occupational testing is in essence a variant of bronchial challenge, but here instead of a measured dose of a purified allergen extract being introduced into the patient, he is exposed to material suspected of causing occupational asthma. Such tests are reserved for material which cannot be quantified, purified and extracted, or when a number of processes are carried out and the allergist does not know which one produces the allergen and which are innocent. The procedure is particularly

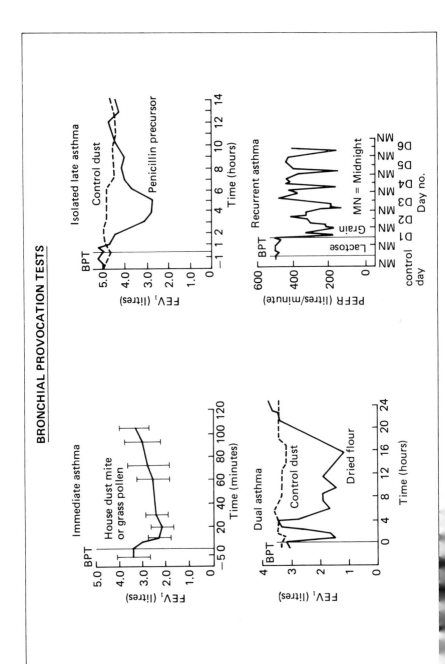

BRONCHIAL PROVOCATION TESTS

Immediate asthma

House dust mite or grass pollen

Dual asthma

Control dust

Dried flour

Isolated late asthma

Control dust

Penicillin precursor

Recurrent asthma

Lactose

Grain

MN = Midnight

BPT

control day

Day no.

D1 D2 D3 D4 D5 D6

FEV₁ (litres)

PEFR (litres/minute)

Time (minutes)

Time (hours)

useful for the evaluation of new allergens. It is carried out in a specially constructed test booth where the patient reproduces as exactly as possible the circumstances of work, and the results are monitored in the same way as in the case of bronchial challenge. The test is, indeed, the same, with the sole difference that the challenge dose cannot be exactly quantified. It should be noted that when an occupational disease has been diagnosed questions of compensation, change of employment and re-training may be involved and thus it is essential that the doctors who carry out such tests shall have sufficient understanding that their opinions will be acceptable to the appropriate government authorities, otherwise the test may need to be repeated by such an accepted person. This, as we have seen above, should never be necessary.

To conclude this part we feel that we must firmly restate the principle that all these tests involve a high risk and should remain solely in the hands of experienced allergists in regular practice. Any delegation that such a responsible person arranges should be by mutual consent and no nurse or technician should be required to undertake duties in this field for which they have not been thoroughly prepared, and about which they feel justified confidence. Such tests should under no circumstances be undertaken unless the allergist is immediately present in the test area throughout the whole time involved.

ELIMINATION DIETING

The remaining category of testing to be considered in this chapter is elimination dieting. This is a much simpler procedure than some of the above and should be in use in all allergy clinics where a full range of diagnostic services is provided. We have seen that prick testing is unreliable for foods and RAST not yet either freely available or of equal validity in all foodstuffs. Thus we turn to a well established technique for diagnosis. The essence of this is that the patient is removed for a test period from all foods which can give rise to problems, during which time significant clinical improvement will occur if food allergy is present. Thereafter individual foods are reintroduced singly in order to measure the occurrence of allergic reactions. All foods are, therefore, eliminated from the diet at one go, but their reintroduction must be separate, in order to measure the response.

Whilst the principle as thus enunciated is simple, the practicalities are not; to carry out this procedure well is one of the most difficult tasks in allergy and is frequently ill performed. It seems to the authors that we are sometimes more scrupulous when the money being spent is on our side of the fence than on the patient's. Clearly this test costs no more to the National Health Service than the production of a leaflet, but the patient is exposed to considerable nuisance and some discomfort. Under these circumstances we owe it to him to ensure that the test is correctly carried out and does not need to be repeated because of errors that could have been avoided.

Elimination dieting is used in a wide-ranging number of allergic problems, including eczema, urticaria, angio-oedema, all respiratory reactions including asthma, gastrointestinal reactions and psychiatric disorders which may include severe psychosis. For this reason the test is not to be lightly undertaken, as a curious phenomenon occurs following an elimination of foods and their re-introduction if they prove to be allergens and that is an increase in the severity of response. Thus a patient may have moderate asthma which improves on elimination, but may develop severe bronchospasm on re-introduction of a trigger food. This possibility should be borne in mind.

The selection of the 'safe' basic diet upon which the whole procedure is based is not without its problems. Probably the only substance which all researchers could agree is safe is distilled water and this has no food value. There are those who do upon occasion use such a draconian regimen for a short period, but this is usually on an in-patient basis on very severe cases. At the least the patient will require time off work during such a fast. Most workers use as a basic diet a compromise which contains a range of foods which clinical experience suggests are only rarely associated with allergy. Such a diet will not merely be a compromise: it may have to be a compromise tailored to the disease process that is being investigated. Thus sugars may be of considerable importance in psychiatric illness, whereas pips are less significant. By contrast, nuts and pips are among the commonest causes of asthma, while sugars cause it but rarely.

Elimination dieting gives rise to the problem that if a large number of foods are removed from the normal pattern of intake a vitamin or mineral deficiency may follow if such a programme is followed for any length of time; this is particularly so in children. In the authors' view no scheme should be pursued for longer than six weeks without at least the support of a dietician to assist with these aspects.

The diets appended are those developed by the author over the past twelve years and are minor modifications of the original McEwen dieting system. Generally the basic diet is used, with most patients able to take either apples or pears, which are only omitted in those known to react unfavourably to them. The same reason forms the only common limitation to the inclusion of mutton or beef, although some subjects who are exquisitely sensitive to milk may react to beef as well. If in doubt the patient should be advised to exclude it. Patients with multiple or psychiatric symptoms should also omit sugar and those with joint and limb pains and general malaise may require to cut out wheat flour and products, including bran. It has been found that patients with gut symptoms who have required bran find sufficient roughage and residue content at least in the short term from buckwheat, to which relatively few British subjects seem to be sensitive. Where an even more limited diet appears to be required the strict diet is used.

The time interval which the patient should spend on either the basic or strict diet varies with different diseases. Some workers have reported conclusive results after intervals of only a few days, but we feel that an interval of at least three weeks is normally required and that for conditions such as eczema and joint pains that four weeks will be essential. In the first fortnight, indeed, the patient may report a worsening of symptoms and may not show improvement until the end of the diet period. For the same reason we prefer that when foods are re-introduced singly into the diet to provoke the recurrence of symptoms the time employed should be seven days. It is not sufficient merely to show improvement when foods are withdrawn. For elimination dieting to have any scientific credibility it is essential that certain foods can also be shown to reproduce the patient's symptoms on challenge, preferably on more than one occasion.

This is a field where a number of variations occur. There is no substitute for learning a satisfactory regimen in a clinic where such procedures are routinely carried out. The subject really requires a whole book. Unfortunately, from the scientific viewpoint, the technique is a tool capable of misuse, producing poor and untrustworthy results, which may undermine the efforts of those who seek to use it to the best advantage of both the patient and professions, so that attention to scientific principles is essential.

Once the method has been learned there is no field in allergy where the common sense and practicality possessed by nurses can be put to better use, as nurses are usually much better at advising on food and its preparation than doctors, whose knowledge of cooking tends to be theoretical rather than practical! Inevitably patients will have a number of time-consuming queries about such diets, which must be borne with great patience if good results are to be achieved; nurses often have more practical experience of cooking than do doctors and may thus be in a better position to give advice. If a trained dietician can be enlisted this represents the ideal for managing this investigation.

Dietary instructions

Before elimination dieting begins the patient should be given a full explanation of what is involved and offered an opportunity to ask questions about any points which are not fully understood. A written sheet of instructions and written notes on dietary restrictions and requirements are essential to ensure that the patient will not become confused about what is allowed and what is not.

A suggested wording for the instruction is given below.

There are no simple tests for food allergy. At present both skin and blood tests are inaccurate and you **cannot rely** on your own judgement either, as it is possible to be allergic to your favourite food or to several foods that you eat every day. This may result in a gradual worsening of symptoms without the true cause being suspected.

The only reliable test is what is called 'elimination dieting'. This consists of spending time (three to four weeks) on a 'safe' diet. If improvement results it is evidence that food allergy is likely to be present. This can be checked by re-introducing foods one at a time for a week each until the culprit is found. This is a medical diagnostic procedure and is best done under specialist supervision, in order to be sure that the results are correct and to ensure that you do not run into health problems, which may happen if dieting is continued for too long. Allergy diets (this one included) are often short of the vitamins and minerals needed for normal healthy living. They should not be followed for more than four weeks without medical advice. If you are asked to omit all cereals from your list you should take a vitamin B supplement. Your chemist can advise you.

Please stick rigidly to the diet and do not try to bend the rules, as a single lapse can sometimes affect the result. If in doubt, *ask*!

These diets are very bland and lack flavour. For variety you may like to try some of the herb beverages available from most health shops. Balm, chamomile, fennel herb, rosemary and yerba mate are allowable, without milk. Dandelion coffee containing dandelion and lactose only is also permissable, made weak and not more than three cups per day.

A number of prepared foods contain substances such as milk or whey. You will have to develop the habit of checking labels. It is possible to check allergy to food additives and preservatives using these diets under medical supervision.

The table on pp. 71–78 shows what is allowed and what is omitted on the basic diet.

Strict allergy exclusion diet

The patient may eat only the following:

> Sugar (brown or white), treacle, golden syrup
> Pearl sago, sago flour, buckwheat, arrowroot
> Lamb, mutton, venison
> Fresh green vegetables, celery, lettuce, carrots, parsnips
>   turnips, up to 6 oz (180 g) per day. No cauliflower,
>   broccoli or spinach
> Tomor margarine (kosher)

Salt
Bicarbonate of soda, cream of tartar
Water, home-made soda water
Tea or tisanes without milk or lemon
Rhubarb, fresh or frozen

As the patient will not be familiar with how to cook using only the very limited variety of items allowed on this list, it is as well to supply some suggested recipes and menus.

Breakfast: Sago savoury cakes fried in Tomor
Sago crispbread with Tomor margarine, treacle or Syrup
Tea without milk or lemon

Mid-morning, afternoon or evening: Tea without milk or lemon, soda water
Sago cakes or shortbread, etc.

Lunch: Vegetable soup
Mutton or lamb
Allowed vegetables
Savoury sago cakes
Sago pudding, rhubarb crumble etc.

Supper: Cold lamb
Salad of celery, green vegetables, lettuce, carrot
Sago crispbread with Tomor
Rhubarb with sugar

Drinks: Tea without milk or lemon
Home-made soda water

Recipes

Potato cakes. Cook 6 oz (180 g) potatoes in salted water until soft. Mash with the Tomor and shape into rounds about 1 in (2.5 cm) thick. Fry in Tomor or bake in the oven at 375°F until golden brown.

Hashed potatoes. Melt Tomor in a frying pan and place in prepared mashed potato, pressing it down. Fry until one side is brown, then turn over and brown the other side.

The basic elimination diet

Omit	Allowed
Milk, whether ordinary, tinned or powdered. Also milk products such as icecream	Carnation brand evaporated milk diluted with water, up to 0.5 pt (0.25 litre) per day
Eggs, chicken or other poultry products or game. Egg products such as custard or salad cream	
Nuts: brazils, hazels, coconuts and nut products such as groundnut oil, some margarines, macaroons	
Beans: chocolate, coffee (fresh or freeze dried or granular varieties such as Nescafe or Gold Blend	Powdered instant coffee (produced by heat precipitation), not more than three weak cups per day
Soya and soya products such as soft margarine, soya mince, soya milk, creamers such as Coffee Compliment and Coffeemate, Marvel, vegetable oils	Hard margarines, preferable Tomor (kosher) or Waitrose Low Fat Spread which is also milk-free
Pulses such as peas, beans, lentils or peanuts (they are not nuts)	
Pips and seeds, as occur in: tomatoes (including juices and ketchups), plums, damsons, cherries, apricots, peaches, prunes, almonds (not a nut; also marzipan and almond paste), apples, pears, strawberries, raspberries, currants (red, black or white), citrus fruits (lemon, orange, grapefruit). All jams, marmalades and other items made from these, including squashes, fruit jellies, sweets, lollies and peppermint. Grapes, sultanas, currants, raisins, figs, dates. Melon, cucumber, marrows, courgettes. Spices such as pepper, mustard or curry powder	Bananas, fresh pineapple, rhubarb (fresh, not frozen or tinned). Some people may have apples and pears (fresh only), but remove the cores before eating or cooking. Tea. If apples are allowed then so is still apple juice
Yeast, as in Marmite, Oxo, Bovril, gravy browning etc. Also occurs in some packet soups and children's tinned meals	Bicarbonate of soda, cream of tartar or baking powder may be used as raising agents

Omit	Allowed

Fish

Cheese

Onions and garlic

Alcohol and vinegar

Meats: pork and bacon. All offal (liver, kidney, tripe, sweetbreads etc.) from any animal	Beef and beef dripping. Rabbit. Mutton, but not small spring lamb. Some people may be allowed beef or mutton but not both

Shellfish

Honey	Sugar is generally allowed. Some people, however, will react to cane sugar, including golden syrup, and/or beet sugar. Tate and Lyle is cane sugar and British Sugar Corporation (Silver Spoon) is beet. Liquid saccharin (Sweetex, Saxin or Hermesetas), but not more than two drops per portion
Fizzy drinks including colas etc. Some people who react to these are reacting to the preservative used (sulphur), which also occurs in wines	Home-made soda water without flavourings
Cereals	Wheat flour and products may be allowed. Make your own soda bread, biscuits and cakes where possible. If bought, no cream, colouring, fruit, nuts, jams or icing Pearl barley. Rye (mostly pumpernickel), though most rye crispbreads contain wheat; Ryeking is one that contains no wheat. Oats (porridge and meal). Rice. Sago. Corn on the cob (maize), including corn oil for cooking and cornflour. Arrowroot. Buckwheat, including buckwheat flour; some buckwheat pasta, available from health food shops, is wheat-free

Omit	Allowed
Miscellaneous	
Chewing gum	
Cauliflower and broccoli	Other green vegetables. Mushrooms, but not more than 4 oz (120 g) per week and then not all at once. Potatoes, including potato flour; but instant potato only if it contains no milk powder: many do. Root vegetables. Salt.

Sauté potatoes. Slice cooked potatoes and fry in Tomor until golden.

Bubble and squeak. Add left-over cooked cabbage to potato and prepare as for hashed potato. Other vegetables may be used with potatoes in a similar way.

Pommes Normandie. Slice potatoes into thin rounds and layer in an oven-proof dish. Cover with milk from the daily allowance and dot with Tomor. Bake in the oven at 375°F for about 1½ hours until golden.

Duchesse potatoes or potato nests. Pipe prepared mashed potatoes into nests or other shapes on a greased baking sheet and place in a hot oven for about 20 minutes.

Green vegetables. Cook in the usual way in salted water.

Lettuce, carrot and celery. Grate carrot, chop celery and shred lettuce and mix to make an attractive salad. When testing has eliminated them, apples or nuts can be added to this basic mixture. Grated cabbage can be substituted for lettuce and makes the mixture more crunchy.

Glazed carrots. Cook sliced carrots in salt water, but when done toss in melted Tomor.

Braised celery. Cut celery into strips and place in an oven-proof dish, dotted with Tomor. Bake until tender, about 1½ hours.

Vegetable soup. Chop two large carrots, two sticks of celery and

8 oz (24 g) of greens and sauté in 1 oz (30 g) Tomor until soft. Add 1½ pt (about 1 litre), and 1 teaspoonful of pearl sago and simmer till tender. Eat as it is or liquidize to make cream soup.

Stuffed cabbage leaves. Cook whole cabbage leaves in hot water until tender, about 10 minutes. Drain and dry on kitchen paper. Prepare chopped vegetables, adding minced left-over meat if available. Flatten the cabbage leaves and put some of the mixture in the middle of each. Fold up like a parcel and place, with the join underneath, into a shallow oven-proof dish. Dot with Tomor and bake in a hot oven until tender, about 1½ hours.

Society layer. Grease an oven-proof dish with Tomor and fill it with layers of minced meat, sliced carrots and grated or chopped cabbage. Dot with Tomor and bake until tender, about 1½ hours. If potatoes are allowed on your diet, they may be used as an alternative, but allow an extra 15 minutes cooking time.

Basic sago shortcrust pastry. Sieve 8 oz (240 g) of sago flour into a bowl with a pinch of salt and rub in 4 oz (120 g) Tomor until it resembles fine breadcrumbs. Add sufficient water to form a soft dough and then use in the normal way.

Meat and vegetable pie. Chop a selection of permitted vegetables and fry in Tomor until tender. Add minced meat or cubed pre-cooked meat and fry for five more minutes. Put into a pie dish and cover with sago shortcrust. Bake for about 30 minutes.

Fruit pie. Cook rhubarb with a little water (and sugar if allowed) and use with sago shortcrust to make a pie in the usual way.

Sago crumble. Prepare the rhubarb as above. Mix 6 oz (180 g) sago flour with 3 oz (90 g) sugar. Rub in 3 oz (90 g) Tomor. Put the rhubarb in an oven-proof dish, spread the crumble mix over the top and dot with Tomor. Bake in a pre-heated oven at 350°F for 20–30 minutes.

Sago shortbread. Cream together 4 oz (120 g) Tomor and 3 oz (90 g) sugar; then fold in 5 oz (150 g) sago flour. Knead into a firm dough and roll out onto a floured surface. Place onto a greased baking sheet or shortbread tin and bake for 20–30 minutes in a pre-heated oven at 325°F. When cool, cut into slices and sprinkle with sugar.

Viennese fancies. Make the mixture as for sago shortbread, but using 4 oz (120 g) of flour for a softer mixture. Work until soft enough to pipe into paper cases using a piping bag or icing tube. Bake about 20–30 minutes until firm to the touch. When cool, sprinkle with sugar.

Sago syrup steamed pudding. Cream together 4 oz (120 g) Tomor and 4 oz (120 g) sugar until light and fluffy. Fold in 8 oz (240 g) sago flour. Add 1 teaspoonful of cream of tartar and half a teaspoonful of baking powder. Add two or three tablespoonfuls of water and form into a dough of soft consistency. Grease a pudding basin and put in three tablespoons of golden syrup. Put the dough on top. Cover tightly and steam for 1½–2 hours. If you do not have a sweet tooth, reduce the amount of sugar by half.

Sago delight. Cook 1½ oz (45 g) of pearl sago in a small amount of water until it has been absorbed and the mixture is stiff. Add 1 oz (30 g) sugar and two tablespoons of syrup. Spread the mixture onto a greased baking sheet and cook for about 30–35 minutes. When cool, cut into squares.

Sago pudding. Place 1½ oz (45 g) pearl sago into a saucepan with half a pint (0.25 litres) Carnation milk and the same amount of water. Bring to the boil and simmer for about 10–15 minutes until cooked through. Serve hot with stewed rhubarb or cold. This pudding can be made in the oven, using the same ingredients but baking at 325°F for two hours until soft and creamy.

Sago coffee pudding. Make as above but add one or two teaspoons of instant coffee to the mixture.

Rhubarb sago pudding. Make in the same way but cook the sago in a thin purée of rhubarb and water instead of Carnation and water.

Crisp-topped caramel sago. Cook in the same way as above. When done, sprinkle with brown sugar and a little melted Tomor and place under a hot grill until crisp.

Carnation cream. Cream together 4 oz (120 g) Tomor and 2 oz (60 g) sugar until light and fluffy. Whisk in a tablespoonful of *hot* water, the one teaspoon of *cold* Carnation milk. Keep whisking until very light and fluffy, adding one tablespoon of water and one of Carnation milk. Use for decoration.

Gravy browning. This can be made by caramelizing sugar in a hot oven. Do not use bought gravy browning as it contains chemicals and yeast.

Savoury spread. Add home-made gravy browning to the juices and fat extracted when roasting meat and thicken with sago flour. Add salt to taste.

9

The Initial Treatment

AVOIDANCE MEASURES

The most effective action, where possible, is to eliminate the offending allergen from the patient's environment. This can be easily effected in some cases, such as the removal of an animal from the house, if that is the problem, or the reduction of moulds in damp rooms by increasing the ventilation and keeping the rooms dry. With other allergens, such as the house dust mite, it is relatively easy, but time-consuming, to reduce the amount of allergen in the air. The best ways of describing these methods are given in the instruction sheet on p. 80, which may be given to patients where applicable. This particular sheet was written by one of the authors for a commercial firm. Other drug companies also issue attractively illustrated pamphlets with the same message. The main advantage of a pamphlet that can be taken away by the patient, is that it can be referred to whenever necessary.

In the case of patients with hay fever or, more specifically, pollen allergy, avoidance measures vary in effect according to the severity of the symptoms. It is certainly advisable for all hay fever sufferers to sleep with their windows closed when the pollen count is high. In fact, when possible, they should stay indoors on days when the pollen count is high and keep windows and doors shut. As hot air rises, bringing pollen with it, patients may get added relief from symptoms by sleeping downstairs. The wearing of tinted glasses when outdoors helps to prevent pollen entering the eyes causing them to irritate and discharge. A holiday by the sea is likely to be more comfortable than a country holiday. It may seem obvious, but patients should be advised *not* to go camping in the pollen season! Also it is not always realized that a holiday in a city is suitable, as such

HOUSEHOLD DUST CAN MAKE YOU ILL

Please note the phrase HOUSEHOLD dust. Not all dust is the same. Factory dust or building dust or garden dust is different. It is usually household dust which causes the problems for most patients.

This is because house dust contains a microscopic mite, the house dust mite, which lives in the dust and feeds on shed human skin scales. This is what makes house dust so different and it is mainly the mite which causes the allergy.

FOR THIS REASON EXTRA CARE IS REQUIRED, ESPECIALLY IN CERTAIN ROOMS AND PLACES.

1) The bed - Your mattress probably has 10 000 mites in it at present! Make a cover from building-grade polythene secured with plastic carpet tape obtainable from any large hardware store. Leave an end open to allow the mattress to ventilate. Vacuum the mattress before you fit the cover and remove the cover about once a month and repeat. Damp dust the mattress cover weekly in between. This removes mites and the skin scales which provide their food. Get rid of feather pillows and replace with a foam type.

Old-fashioned eiderdowns and duvets filled with feathers can cause problems and should be disposed of. However, if covers are really featherproof and you are not allergic to feathers you may be all right. Duvets filled with synthetic materials are satisfactory. Don't use NYLON sheets - they carry a static electric charge and attract dust. Cotton cellular blankets are best. Blankets should be washed and aired frequently.

2) The bedroom - People with this problem usually improve in hospital as wards are designed to minimise dust traps. Arrange your bedroom to be without dust traps as far as possible. Keep furnishings as light and simple as you can.

3) The rest of the house - Damp dust and vacuum clean. Get someone else to empty vacuum bags. DO NOT BRUSH CARPETS AND FURNITURE. Avoid paraffin heaters which make for a damp house. Dust mites like damp houses.

4) On holiday - A rarely used spare bedroom will contain more mites than one used constantly. If you are to use one try to have it thoroughly cleaned before use. You may need to take some bedding (pillows, etc.) with you.

Sleeping bags should be thoroughly aired and cleaned before you go camping as they can accumulate a lot of mites when stored in a cupboard from year to year.

THE ANSWER TO HOUSE DUST ALLERGY IS MAINLY
HOUSEWORK. INJECTIONS MAY BE SOME HELP,
BUT ONLY IN ADDITION TO THE ABOVE, NOT INSTEAD.

areas are also relatively low in pollen. Commercially produced leaflets are also available to cover this field of advice.

None of these measures, however, will bring complete relief except to very mildly sensitive patients: therefore, others will require different forms of treatment.

DRUG THERAPY

Antihistamines

You will recall that in Chapter 3 histamine release was discussed. Clearly antihistamine drugs inhibit histamine release at the site of inflammation or allergic reaction. Antihistamines may be sufficient to relieve symptoms completely or alleviate them to a large extent. Thus for some patients no other treatment will be needed. They are also very useful in the treatment of patients who present too late for desensitization to take place before the hay fever season starts and may also be given during the period of desensitization if required.

There are some side effects to these drugs, the most important being that they may induce drowsiness and patients who drive cars or operate machinery may not be able to take them. It will, no doubt, come as a surprise to you to learn that almost all antihistamine tablets may be purchased from a pharmacist, without a prescription. Many people do buy the tablets after describing their problem to the pharmacist as either runny or blocked nose or runny and itching eyes etc. The choice of tablets is governed, to a large extent, by the cost. Some preparations recommended for the treatment of hay fever symptoms are very expensive. An example is Rynacrom Nasal Spray (sodium cromoglycate) at approximately £5.45 at the time of writing.

The table on p. 82 lists antihistamines that may be purchased without a prescription from a chemist providing the sale is negotiated by a dispensing pharmacist. Under these circumstances trade names are generally used, but approved names are also given.

One drug which is marketed as an antihistamine, however, has additional properties claimed for it: this is azatadine

Antihistamine preparations

Brand name	Approved name	Remarks
Available without prescription		
Actidil	triprolidine hydrochloride	
Anthisan	mepyramine maleate	
Benadryl SA	diphenhydramine hydrochloride	
Daneral SA	pheniramine maleate	
Dimotane LA	brompheniramine maleate	
Dimotapp LA	brompheniramine maleate/ phenylephrine hydrochloride/ phenylpropanolamide	Frequently recommended by chemists
Fabahistin	mebhydrolin	Widely used
Fenostil Retard	dimethindene maleate	
Haymine	chlorpheniramine maleate/ ephedrine hydrochloride	
Histryl	diphenylpyraline	
Lergoban	diphenylpyraline	
Periactin	cyproheptadine hydrochloride	
Phenergan	promethazine hydrochloride	Cheapest, but has sedative action; useful at night
Piriton	chlorpheniramine maleate	Cheap. Well known and widely used
Pro-Actidil	triprolidine hydrochloride	
Tavegil	clemastine	
Thephorin	phenindamine tartrate	
Available on prescription only		
Banistyl	dimethothiazine mesylate	
Optimine	azatadine maleate	
Primalan	mequitazine	
Vallergan	trimeprazine tartrate	

maleate (Optimine). It is claimed that it is also a serotonin antagonist. We have met serotonin before in Chapter 3 as one of the other mediators of allergy. This is the first drug which is claimed to have an action on these other mediators, but it is unlikely to be the last. Furthermore, we now know that histamine itself is secreted in two forms, H_1 and H_2, and that it is H_2 which is secreted in the lungs. This is why antihistamines do not have any effect when administered for asthma, because they are H_1 antagonists. Recently an H_2 antagonist cimetidine (Tagamet) has been marketed for use in gastric ulceration, where H_2 is also secreted. The place of this drug in allergy has yet to be fully evaluated, but at the time of writing its chief use in the authors' hands is in urticaria, but it is not to be considered as a drug of first choice. Like most newer preparations it is exceedingly expensive, especially in a therapeutic dose which is usually high.

It should be noted that all antihistamines *inhibit skin test reactivity* and patients attending for an allergy consultation should be warned to cease their use at the very least 48 hours before testing and preferably five days before their appointment. In general practice this warning can be administered verbally, but in hospital clinics it should be sent out with the appointment card. It is necessary to warn patients that drugs such as cough mixtures are extremely likely to contain antihistamines. At the same time they should be advised *not* to stop essential anti-asthmatics such as steroids or DSCG which have no effect on immediate skin test reactivity. Bronchodilators such as salbutamol are probably innocent of major effects on skin testing, but there is some variation of opinion on this.

Other drugs

Some other substances often used in the treatment of allergy symptoms are shown on p. 89. A number of these are *decongestants*.

Many of the topical nasal decongestants which are marketed to the general public have the disadvantage of producing the phenomenon known as *rebound congestion*. Initially, the action of a decongestant is to produce vasoconstriction in the small

Other drugs used in treatment of allergy

Brand name	Approved name
Available without prescription	
Antistin-Privine	antazoline sulphate/naphthazoline
Eskornade	isopropamide/phenylpropanolamine/ diphenylpyraline
Intal	sodium cromoglycate
Otrivine	xylometazoline hydrochloride
Rynacrom	sodium cromoglycate
Triominic	phenylpropanolamine/mepyramine maleate/ pheniramine maleate
Available on prescription only	
Dexa-Rhinaspray	tramazoline hydrochloride
Non-ethicals (off prescription only)	
Do-Do Tablets	
Fenox	
Mucron	
Sinex	

blood vessels of the nose. As the therapeutic effect wears off it is natural to expect that vasoconstriction will return to normal. In fact it does not: active vasodilatation takes place. This has the effect of making the nasal obstruction of the sufferer worse than it was before treatment and therefore there is usually a further recourse to the decongestant. This time it wears off even more quickly and thus in a chronic nasal condition the patient may eventually be left with a nasal obstruction which is virtually complete in spite of the use of the drops or spray in a dose far in excess of that recommended by the manufacturer. It is common to find that in many patients presenting to ENT surgeons little, if any, treatment is required other than to stop the use of these preparations. Like such surgeons the authors deprecate the use of these substances, some of which are prescribable, especially since there are safer alternatives available.

Disodium cromoglycate (sodium cromoglycate, DSCG, SCG, or cromolyn sulfate), a fascinating and extremely valuable drug, has been available since 1967 when it was first introduced in the United Kingdom. It is now marketed in a number of forms for use in allergic disorders and is available as eyedrops, nasal drops and spray, 'Spinhaler' inhalation capsules for thoracic use and capsules for use in bowel disorders. It is extremely well tolerated with very few side effects and is of extremely low toxicity. Without any doubt this is one of the few drugs to which the term 'breakthrough' might fairly be applied; for many allergic sufferers it has represented a revolution in treatment and provided adequate relief from symptoms for the first time. At one time it was even suggested that treatments such as this were going to put the allergist out of a job. However, this has not proved to be the case and we should briefly consider the reasons. The first is that its action is not usually prolonged. We do not know the precise pharmacological mode of action of the drug, in spite of a great deal of research, but in very simple terms it may be said to 'coat' the mast cell and thereby help to prevent mast cell degranulation (see Chapter 3). Any 'coating' applied to living tissue does not remain and therefore the dose needs to be repeated. This means that disodium cromoglycate must be taken preventively and regularly if it is to work effectively. For most patients this will mean three or four times daily and in children sometimes more frequently. Not all patients, particularly children, are willing or able to do this. Secondly some patients do not respond to the drug. We do not know why this should be, as they do not seem in any way to be an identifiable or distinct group. The third problem with disodium cromoglycate is cost. It is inappropriate to give a precise figure for this in a textbook, but referral to MIMS will give you the current figure. If one reflects that some patients will need eye, nose and chest treatment continuously for years on end to remain symptom-free it will be seen that the cost of such therapy, especially to the National Health Service, is very considerable. In the view of the authors, therefore, such treatment should be used only when simpler treatment is ineffective and its long-term use should be reserved for cases where no prospect exists of reducing the patient's need for treatment.

Ketotifen (Zaditen) is a new preparation which has become available on the United Kingdom Market since September 1979. Although chemically unrelated to disodium cromoglycate, it is claimed to have a 'cromon-like', i.e. similar, action in stabilizing mast cells and can thus be used on a regular basis to ward off attacks. It is known to have an antihistamine-like action and it is also said to be anti-anaphylactic, which is not the same thing. Unlike DSCG, it is administered by mouth. On theoretical grounds it obviously offers considerable prospects of being a useful addition to our range of available palliatives, not only for asthma, but possibly for rhinitis, ophthalmia and maybe even intestinal and skin manifestations of allergy. It is an expensive preparation, but if it can be used to control more than one aspect of allergy, the cost will then become more moderate. Papers are now beginning to emerge showing efficacy in rhinitis and urticaria and other skin diseases in addition to its primary use in asthma, for which it was originally offered. It may also be of value in some cases of food allergy. Because of this wide range of use it should be considered in all cases where multiple symptoms of allergy are experienced.

The *steroids* comprise a large group of preparations related in chemical structure and action to cortisol, but usually showing enhanced potency. The place for a detailed discussion of their mode of action lies in a pharmacology rather than an allergy textbook and suitable references will be found at the end of this book.

The use for which steroids have been best known for the longest period is systemically, as in asthma. Although cortisone can be used, it is usual to employ artificial steroid drugs such as prednisolone or prednisone. These have a potency five times greater than cortisone itself in its various forms. Most of the other orally administered steroids have a similar enhanced potency: because of this they have a potential not only for good, but also for harmful side effects. These are very well known, but will bear repeating. They include the development of Cushing's syndrome, osteoporosis, diabetes mellitus, skin atrophy and suprarenal insufficiency; because of this it has always been considered proper to restrict their use to conditions where the severity of the condition warrants such major treatment. Precisely the same objection applies to the use of systemically acting depot steroids, which are normally either methylprednisolone acetate or triamcinolone acetamide (marketed respectively as Depo-Medrone or Kenalog). Unfortunately these preparations are used with much greater freedom as there seems to be a much less acute awareness of the problems they can engender. Exactly the same precautions should be taken with regard to the issuing of steroid cards as if the patient was on any other steroid treatment. Depot steroids are not infrequently used in hay fever, as a single injection at the start of the season. In the authors' view, if it is felt that the hay fever is sufficiently severe to warrant the use of steroid therapy it is preferable to use a preparation such as prednisolone because of its increased dosage flexibility; the risks are the same and no greater.

At times steroids themselves have been replaced by ACTH (adrenocorticotrophic hormone). This stimulates natural cortisol secretion and is therefore devoid of the risk of inducing suprarenal insufficiency, although pituitary suppression may obviously occur. The other risks of ACTH are the same as for any other mode of delivering steroids. There is an additional risk, as these hormones are either derived from animal sources, and contain some foreign protein, or synthetically produced, but still foreign protein. Both are potential and actual sensitizers, especially in allergic patients. The advantages are a once or twice weekly dosage schedule and the administration being kept under medical and nursing care because ACTH can be administered only by injection.

Steroids have also been used for many years in topical therapy on skin and in mucous membranes. Earlier types of topical steroid were identical to those used orally and were found to be systemically absorbed from the site of application. This can be important when the patient is an infant or small child, for instance when large areas of the body are covered by an anxious and poorly informed mother, or even in adults where large areas of the body are treated for a considerable period of time, as in psoriasis. Because of this, much work has been done to produce topical steroids which are not generally absorbed, and thus this effect may be reduced. However, the skin atrophy produced by long-term steroids still remains and as some of these newer forms are more potent can occasionally be a worse problem than the original allergy.

The use of such non-absorbed steroids has led to a development of very considerable value in inhalant allergy, which is to deliver to the site of allergy a non-absorbed steroid, thus providing a potent anti-allergic effect at the site of response whilst minimizing the generalized effects. Both beclomethasone dipropionate and beclomethasone valerate have been used and are available as metered aerosols, the former for thoracic and nasal applications and the latter for thoracic only. Since the introduction of these two, flunisolide has also been marketed for nasal use. This step constitutes another revolution, especially in the treatment of childhood asthma, where formerly the clinician was reluctant to use systemic steroids but felt that the patient needed more potent treatment than he or she was receiving. Earlier fears that fungal overgrowth or atrophy would occur have been shown to be mostly unfounded and these preparations are now used freely. The one practical disadvantage is that they are not absorbed when a free mucus secretion is present and in exacerbations may need to be replaced by a short course of oral steroids or ACTH. In practice many steroid-dependent patients have been weaned off their systemic therapy onto these drugs with consequent improvement in their general health. Although not as expensive as DSCG, these preparations are not cheap and you may wish at this point to remind yourself of the current cost of treatment.

Many topical treatments can be purchased from the chemist without a prescription. Some are listed on p. 89. Anthisan and Caladryl are antihistamines. Used topically these are regarded by most dermatologists as sensitizers and their use is strongly deprecated by most doctors in this specialty. The objection to Caladryl does not apply to calamine lotion or cream itself, which contains no antihistamine.

All steroid preparations are only available on a doctor's

Topical treatments for allergy

Brand name	Approved name
	hypromellose
Anthisan	mepyramine maleate
Caladryl	calamine/camphor/diphenhydramine hydro- chloride
	calamine
Eurax	crotamiton
E45 Cream	
Parfenac	bufexamac
Ultrabase	
Unguentum Merck	

prescription. There are a number of non-steroid skin treatments which can be prescribed instead. They include E45, Parfenac, Unguentum Merck and Ultrabase. These are used when a steroid is not required and in the authors' view drugs of this sort are as underused as the steroids are over-prescribed.

10

Hyposensitization

We must now move on to the most vital aspect of a book on allergy, which is to consider the treatment which is peculiar to allergy and which, in most instances, can be provided only by an allergist, and then only after the processes previously discussed.

In Chapter 3 we considered, among other things, the nature of blocking antibody. We must now consider this substance in relation to hyposensitization.

We have seen that in the allergic patient the reaction between the allergen and patient results in the formation of IgE antibody, which is what causes release of the mediators of allergy. We have seen that in the non-allergic, non-atopic (Pepys) patient the reaction with allergen to form IgE does not take place. Such a reaction does occur in the untreated allergic patient who will have a high specific IgE for the allergen concerned. This raised level may fluctuate at different times of year, especially for seasonal allergens; in this case it is at a raised level pre-seasonally as compared with normal, but reaches its peak at the point of maximum contact with the allergen, e.g. a hay fever patient will achieve this peak in June and July. After the season the level will fall gradually to the pre-seasonal level. In the treated patient, where allergen extracts are given pre-seasonally, there is an initial rise in IgE, but not to the height attained by a seasonal peak. This is followed by a fall in titre to a lower level than before, but this low level may rise during the season, although the increase does not reach the normal peak, and instead usually attains the pre-seasonal level. In a patient fully treated there may be no rise in IgE in the season. This is the stage at which our postulated blocking antibody is considered to be at its maximum.

However, this reaction is, of course, molecule by molecule; for example, when the patient has received only a small amount of allergen by injection, and is then exposed to a large amount of the same allergen occurring naturally, he may be at first protected and then experience a breakthrough of symptoms as his blocking antibody is exhausted. This is why the patient with hay fever may be satisfactorily controlled after treatment in a mild season, but if the pollen count is high may experience symptoms. Clearly if the dose of pollen is sufficient, and the blocking antibody exhausted, the hay fever may in that year be as bad as before treatment. Equally, it should be clear that the rate at which the body can react to a dose of allergen by blocking antibody formation will be finite; a very heavy dose of injected allergen may be sufficient to allow enough free circulating material to reach the site of allergy; IgE release will then take place, with the consequent appearance of symptoms. This thus limits the rate at which allergen can be given in a hyposensitizing course.

Thus there is a need to determine the dose which will produce an immune state, without inducing allergy. Although this can now be studied by modern immunological techniques, the courses that we are using were, in fact, originated by entirely empirical methods very many years ago; by and large the current emphasis does not seem to suggest that a total revision of these will be necessary. When such techniques eventually pass into routine clinical work it is probable that our existing units of measurement of allergic activity will be superceded by a direct measurement of allergic potential, but until then two systems of measurement are employed. The oldest, which was referred to in Chapter 1 is the *noon unit*. This is defined as 1 millionth of a gram (10^{-6} g) of pollen or other allergen in 1 ml of solution.

This unit is still in use by one of the three firms marketing allergy products in the United Kingdom (Bencard). The newer unit is the *protein nitrogen unit* (PNU). This is defined as 0.00001 mg of protein nitrogen. This unit is used by the other two firms in the field. Although a rough unofficial unit of conversion exists, it is considered to be inexact as the two systems do not measure exactly the same thing. Thus you will not find it in this book and the authors do not consider that its use should be encouraged.

HYPOSENSITIZATION

In general, if a patient has received treatment using one system, and is to receive the other next year, make no assumptions.

HYPOSENSITIZING SOLUTIONS

The types of solution available must now engage our attention. Although skin testing extracts are glycerinated, such materials are not used in hyposensitization, as oily substances have been reported as carcinogens. Thus the basic form of allergy injections is in normal saline. These are the oldest type of injection and are in essence similar in principle to those used by Noon in 1911, although it has been found possible with clinical experience to reduce the total number of injections to 18 per course. Such materials are marketed by Bencard as *specific desensitizing vaccine* (SDV). The whole range of skin test solutions marketed by this firm is available as SDV, either singly or in combination. These extracts are not standardized but must be prescribed individually for each patient; an order form available from the company is required with each prescription before it can be dispensed. A common procedure is the administration of *maintenance therapy*, which is a process whereby the final dose reached in *initial* treatment is repeated at a set interval, usually one month, in order to maintain and perhaps enhance the IgG antibody level reached. SDV maintenance sets are available on the same basis. When such an extract is required it is of assistance to the company if it is prescribed at the same time as the initial treatment set; if not, the company's reference should be quoted to enable them, where possible, to ensure that both come from the same batch of material if available, although this may clearly not be possible from one year to the next. This principle clearly holds good for all specific extracts from any company.

SDV is an invaluable product which has stood the test of time and is still in regular use. However, it does require a large number of injections and because of this attempts have been made to find a means of dispensing a material which reduces the total number required. Such procedures involve some form of combination of the allergen with other material to promote a slow release of allergen, thus enabling a larger amount to be given in a single dose without risk of IgE breakthrough. One such product formerly marketed was D.Vac which was oil-based. This gave good results with a minimal number of injections, but for a number of reasons has not been available for many years. However, as patients may refer to it you should be aware of its former existence.

The combination in greatest use at present is *aluminium adsorption*, where the allergen is attached onto an alum base. This achieves a slow release and allows the number of injections to be reduced to nine or ten per course. You should note that the allergen is **ad**sorbed *onto* the alum, not **ab**sorbed *into* it: hence it is easily detachable in the body to enable IgG synthesis to take place. Extracts based on this principle are marketed by all three firms. Bencard do not make their entire range available in this form (a few are available only as SDV), but for both the other firms, who only offer alum-precipitated vaccines, the complete range is obviously available in this format. The Bencard range consists of Alavac P. which is a standard extract of grass pollen alone, containing all 12 of the most common (see Chapter 4). This can be prescribed without a special order form and is intended for pre-seasonal treatment of hay fever. Alavac S is a range of specific vaccines, made to the individual requirements of the patient and requiring an order form. Dome Laboratories offer two vaccines, Allpyral G, which is an equivalent to Alavac S and used in the same way for the same indications but containing five grass pollens, and Allpyral S, which is similar in availability and usage to Alavac S. There is, however, one difference, as the manufacturer recommends that extracts of house dust mite should not be combined with any other allergen. Merck offer Norisen Grass, similar to the other standard grass mixes but this time containing six grass pollens, and Norisen, which is their specific range. As with Alavac all their extracts can be mixed. All three firms offer maintenance therapy courses in this format.

There are occasions when a patient is assessed as having extreme sensitivity to an allergen and the allergist needs to start with an extremely low dose. Under these circumstances all three manufacturers in the field can supply what is called a special dilution vial, with a strength of 10 PNU/ml: the usual starting strength is 100 PNU/ml. A suitable number of injections from this lower strength then precede the dosage on the first vial.

The remaining manoeuvre to simplify allergen administration available in the United Kingdom at present is to combine the allergen with *tyrosine* which is an essential amino acid; this has enabled two shorter courses to be marketed, both by Bencard. These are both standardized extracts. Pollinex is a three-dose course for the treatment of hay fever pre-seasonally and Migen a six-dose course for the treatment of house dust mite allergy. Both can be prescribed directly without an order form.

You have seen that throughout this chapter we have referred to pre-seasonal treatment of hay fever and the question of timing in relation to treatment must next be considered. Perennial allergens may all be administered at any time of year, but pollens are not given during their pollination period, as the effect of a dose given by injection when the patient is already suffering may well be to induce an intense allergy, or even an anaphylactic reaction. In the past what were termed *co-seasonal* courses were available from Bencard and Dome, but these have now been withdrawn as they have enjoyed very limited support in recent years. All pollen courses are now given before their flowering season; ideally the course should commence so that the last dose is given one month before the season commences and no later. If a course finishes much before this it is usual to repeat the last dose weekly until one month before the expected date of the pollen season.

Extracts of stinging insects are a special group. They should never under any circumstances be mixed with any other extract and should always be given before the season, with due care because of their potential for anaphylaxis. If the patient is highly sensitized most clinics prefer to start the course in the clinic, handing over to the general practitioner only when it is clear that the patient is responding satisfactorily.

In our view the *venom extracts*, which are new, should remain in the hands of allergists working from well equipped hospital centres with good facilities for resuscitation. Most such allergists, at the present time, prefer to admit the patient as a day case.

The dosage normally has to be determined individually and the allergist will return the patient to the general practitioner or his nurse for maintenance therapy when he is satisfied that a stable state has been achieved. Even at this stage reactions may occur, particularly if the injection coincides with a new sting, and the practitioner and his nurse should check carefully on each occasion that they are happy to give the further injections before accepting this responsibility. Venom extracts offer potent material and we are all anxious that the reputation of this approach should be built up by a responsible policy in these early stages, until the procedure has become well standardized.

PROCEDURE

The ideal situation for the administration of desensitizing injections is during a special session held regularly at the general practitioner's premises with a general practitioner in attendance. Dosages and reactions to be checked are specific to allergy and it is, therefore, easier to maintain the progress of these patients if they are seen on a sessional basis.

The injections are normally given deeply subcutaneously into the upper arm in the deltoid region. They should not be given intradermally. As you may know, when some vaccines for travel abroad are given by such a route the dose is reduced to one-fifth. Inadvertent intradermal administration of allergen extracts would thus be expected markedly to increase the likelihood of anaphylaxis. It is also imperative to remember that the injection must not be given into a blood vessel.

After each dose has been administered the patient must wait until the doctor is satisfied that the risk of anaphylaxis is past, usually ten to twenty minutes. As the doses being administered are small, of the order of 0.05 ml, it is essential that a careful check is made before each dose is given. The patient should be asked if any symptoms of allergy occurred following the last injection, before the next is drawn up, and if there are any systemic reactions or any marked increase in local reactions, the nurse should refer to the doctor. In this situation the last dose will normally be repeated or a return may be made to a lower dose which was experienced without symptoms. Thereafter, dosage next time proceeds in the same way as long as no further symptoms of allergy occur. No return is made to a higher dose missing intermediate steps. It is of no use, if a patient experiences such symptoms, delaying treatment by one week or more and then proceeding to a higher dose. If anything this increases the chances of anaphylaxis. Companies marketing allergy extracts warn that the risks are increased at times when the patient has an infection. However, the same problem will arise if the treatment is stopped totally for two or three weeks and the authors prefer to give a lower safe dose rather than abandon a course unless a patient is seriously ill. Once the course has been stopped, it becomes necessary to start again at the beginning and pre-seasonally there is often insufficient time to do this.

Of the processes involved in allergy work it is the administration of extracts which over the years has caused most of the anaphylactic reactions which have been seen, although in the authors' view most such episodes can be prevented by careful prescribing and administration. Many anaphylactic reactions reported to hospital clinics are from what one might term 'pilot error'.

Any nurse who administers hyposensitizing injections should make sure that the supervising doctor is fully prepared to take responsibility for all her actions, even those that are undertaken in his absence. In particular the actions which the nurse may take if anaphylaxis occurs must be clearly agreed in advance, both with the responsible doctor and with the nurse's employer; such agreements should preferably be recorded in writing. Without such safeguards the legal position of both doctor and nurse in the event of complications is extremely vulnerable. Unless the policy document allows the nurse to administer adrenaline without first calling a doctor, in the opinion of the authors no nurse should agree to carry out desensitizing injections.

Normally nurses are allowed to give adrenaline according to an agreed schedule, but will frequently be required to have ready such substances as injectable steroids or antihistamines for the doctor to administer. As these substances are prepared each time, but thankfully infrequently used, careful checking of the expiry date must be a routine procedure.

Hyposensitization for food allergy has been explored by various workers in the past. Frankland has desensitized patients with single food allergies using a rush desensitization method on an in-patient basis. However, this technique has not been explored further and since many patients have multiple food allergies it may well be that it would not be appropriate to do so. Two techniques are currently in use. The clinical ecologists use extracts produced to a dosage level, that is calculated to what is called the neutralization point. Following the work of Rinkel, it has been found that, shortly after exposure to an allergen to which they are sensitized, some patients will be unreactive. Therefore, a small dose of allergen administered prior to ingestion of a food may enable a dose of a food to which the patient is sensitive to be successfully tolerated. This type of treatment has been carried out on a limited basis both in the United States and in the United Kingdom. Much further work needs to be done on it but one of the authors has seen patients who have undoubtedly shown improvement in clinical symptoms when this type of therapy has been exploited. The other type of treatment now available for food allergies results from the work of Dr L.M. McEwen and is known as enzyme-potentiated transepidermal hyposensitization. This technique exploits the potentiating effect of the enzymes betaglucuronidase and chondroitin sulphate when added to dilute allergen mixtures. One author has personal experience of this technique which is not, as yet, available on the National Health Service. However, the existence of methods that assist with the dreadful problem of food allergies should give us encouragement to realize that we have by no means reached the end of the road in developing hyposensitization techniques.

When due care is taken by all parties involved, the process of hyposensitization is usually uneventful, but such success is achieved only by constant awareness and vigilance, which must never over the years be allowed to slacken.

11

The Allergy Team

The need for a chapter on this subject has grown out of the changes which are taking place in health care in our increasingly technically oriented society. In past years the doctor was inclined to regard himself as sole master of his clinical responsibilities, offering deference to no one else and with the authority to command all members of staff to carry out any orders he might think fit, in the confident expectation that they would be obeyed. Today doctors have had to adapt themselves to a far more democratic and cooperative approach to the patient. Many tiers of lay health service managers regulate the buildings in which both doctors and paramedical staff work and determine contracts of employment and terms and conditions of service. Junior doctors and colleagues in other paramedical disciplines are no longer hand-maidens to consultants, but professions in their own right, subject to detailed academic and practical training. Together with the medical staff, they provide a sophisticated service to the patient, of a kind not dreamed of previously. All those capable of completing such training are likely to have the intellectual capacity to evaluate their role in the team effectively; their views are worth listening to, for all those in the team share the common objective of providing the best possible patient care in the circumstances in which we work.

Nurses in particular now have a precise view of their role in health care and its value. Certain duties have been accepted as traditional, while others are seen as part of the extended role of the nurse. These duties may be carried out with enthusiasm by a nurse who has received the relevant training, and who thus feels confident of her own abilities, but the decision to take on such duties must be an individual one by the nurse concerned. The busy doctor may well seek to utilize nursing colleagues to provide a service in the field of allergy, but this must be with their cooperation and not by compulsion. Most of the duties involved in allergy work, however, do involve some extension of the nurse's traditional role. Nurses are, quite rightly, averse to being used as substitute doctors; they are becoming more aware of the functions and attitudes that are peculiar to nursing and wish to take advantage of the opportunities to do what they do best, i.e. to help the patient manage his problems in the best possible way. We must now discuss the implications of this.

The attitude to patient management exemplified by the term 'the nursing process' is discussed more fully in Chapter 12. Any doctor or paramedical worker, or even nurse, to whom the concept is a new one, should study this chapter with care, as the ideas have much to offer and demand a systematic and constructive approach to the patient. In the out-patient clinic, the practical implications are that the nurse must be given some independent opportunity to follow a patient's path through the clinic so that an assessment of needs can be made, a plan of action carried through and finally appropriate advice arranged. The nurse may need to take responsibility for contacting her colleagues, such as district nurses, to ensure follow-up.

Let us look at a practical example. A child of immigrant origin attends the clinic as a patient. He does speak English, but since he is only young he cannot grasp very complicated instructions. He is accompanied by his mother, who speaks no English and has not acquired, to any significant extent, British cultural attitudes. The diagnosis is house dust mite allergy and it is decided that the problem shall be dealt with initially by a programme of house dust control in the home (see Chapter 9). Under these circumstances, giving a leaflet to either mother or child is unlikely to be effective; further advice, perhaps in the home, from a district nurse or health visitor, will probably be required to ensure understanding and compliance, and hence successful treatment. Such a programme of advice and follow-up is not usually carried out effectively by the doctor and a team effort is involved, with the nurse playing a full part. If such interchanges are to be facilitated, some alterations may be needed in the way doctors structure their clinics.

It can be valuable and convenient to use the clinic nurse for history-taking, but if such a history is to form the basis for testing and subsequent medical treatment, the nurse is extending her traditional role and should do so only under conditions of mutual trust and where proper support is offered to her. Records compiled by the nurse in these circumstances are part of the diagnostic process of the allergy clinic and have a permanent place in the clinic records. They are as confidential as any other medical record. Nurses, like doctors, as professional persons, can be sued or removed from the register for improper activities; she must, therefore, be allowed to make notes, and retain copies if necessary, relating to her activities, especially where these may lead to the implementation of treatment.

The same applies, of course, to skin testing. Allergen extracts are covered by the Medicines Act 1968 under the POM category, which means they can be prescribed only by a physician. Such drugs can be acquired and used by a nurse only when she is working under the clinical direction of a doctor. The doctor concerned must satisfy himself as to the clinical capabilities of the nurse and be prepared to take legal responsibility for her actions. Unless he is so satisfied, he could be regarded as guilty of professional misconduct. In the same way, a nurse who implements treatment without such an understanding from the supervising doctor is laying herself open to legal repercussions. The use of allergen extracts can rarely result in reaction, even anaphylaxis, and no nurse should undertake testing without an agreed emergency procedure and genuine medical cover available at the time of the test.

When the history and skin testing have been completed, a diagnosis will be made. It is universally accepted that this diagnosis is a medical matter, especially since it may lead to a course of injections. Writing out a form for a set of hyposensitizing injections is, in essence, a prescription; the covering form FP10, which results in a NHS prescription, will read 'XYZ make injection course as per order form' and it is only the order form which allows the prescription to be dispensed by the chemist. Consequently it is not reasonable for a doctor to ask a nurse to see patients, conduct skin tests and fill in the order forms on her own, leaving them for the doctor to cover with an enabling prescription at a later date. We have heard of such arrangements, but they are not to be condoned; no health authority will back such programmes when they become officially known. When planning clinic facilities such schemes are not to be contemplated.

Most hyposensitizing injections are in fact carried out in general practice and a similar problem of cover arises. Once again, no nurse should conduct injections without adequate medical cover; in practice this means a doctor, on the premises, who has agreed to assist whenever required. The nurse should have a written policy indicating which emergency drugs, if any, she may administer and under what circumstances. Such drugs must be provided and must be prepared before any injections are given. Most district nurses working for area health authorities have a policy document on these lines, but practice nurses employed directly by a doctor may not. One should be provided and the AHA is usually happy to advise on the terminology.

In a number of clinics, particularly chest ones, the respiratory physiology technicians may assist in clinic work in addition to performing respiratory measurements. The technician will possess a much greater depth of knowledge, in his particular sphere, than will a nurse; but this knowledge is within a much narrower confine and likely to be technical rather than patient-centred. He may therefore be completely unfamiliar with aspects of medicine which would be well known even to a student nurse. For this reason the technician must be regarded as having a role of his own, and not as being a substitute for a nurse.

A qualified respiratory function technician should be able to undertake, in addition to respiratory and blood gas measurements, skin testing and challenge testing. Because of the nature of the technician's training he may need more instruction than a nurse on the skills of history-taking and patient management; it should be agreed in advance what form of history-taking should be employed and what features of it should lead to consultation with a doctor. No technician should be expected to take an allergy history, let alone to initiate skin testing, without an agreement of this nature. The authorization of a technician to use skin testing extracts follows the same lines as authorization for a nurse to do so. The best guidelines in these circumstances are a competently and clearly written job description, acceptable to the consultant, the technician and the technician's professional body. On accepting employment the technician is asked to accept the job description and is then insured by the health authority to carry out the designated procedures. He will probably not be insured for procedures not specifically included in the description. If the consultant wishes to extend the technician's responsibilities he should do so officially in writing by adding to the job description. Otherwise the technician may be at risk of legal action and the doctor may be open to charges of professional misconduct, in that he delegated work to an unqualified person.

Some technicians have no formal qualifications but have been granted a certificate of competence by a consultant at some time in the past. Those entering the profession nowadays will generally seek an O Tech or HNC in the appropriate subject and/or membership of a professional body. In the event of any medicolegal problems it will be helpful to establish that the competence of the technician has been assessed by an independent body; problems might be exacerbated if it could be shown that fitness to practice has not been so assessed. It is clearly wise to encourage those now entering the profession to seek appropriate qualifications. Allergy diagnosis should only be attempted by qualified personnel, never by unsupervised or unqualified students.

One further potential member of the allergy team deserves mention here: the representative of drug manufacturers, whether or not medically or otherwise qualified. For a number of historical reasons it has in the past been the practice for the allergy firms to provide and fund a diagnostic service in allergy. Provided this is staffed by adequately qualified persons, there can be no objections, but it must be made clear on what terms and conditions the service is offered. Is a charge to be made, and if so to whom? Will a comprehensive range of material be available or will the advice given be based on the products of only one firm? If the service is to be offered in a general practitioner's surgery or hospital out-patient department, the doctor must appreciate that he is delegating part of his diagnostic task and once again he must satisfy himself that the person concerned is qualified and has appropriate medical cover and that clinical contact will be sufficient to ensure safe diagnosis and adequate transfer of information. Appropriate medical notes must be made, particularly if a prescription is to result. As we said before, the doctor must be clear that he understands what has been recommended on the order form before authorizing the enabling prescription. If the service is provided in a diagnostic clinic to be passed on to a general practitioner, the latter must ensure that he is supplied with all relevant information before he issues any prescription. Doctors and nurses should refuse to be parties to any arrangement which does not possess satisfactory safeguards.

However, sometimes the service offered will be provided by a person who is, in essence, a pharmaceutical representative who has been given special training by his employers. Such representatives are not required by law to possess a qualification in any of the medical or ancilliary professions and their training is not monitored by any outside body. Such a representative should therefore be regarded, at best, as a very junior technician; the doctor who collaborates with him will clearly, for his own safety, have to provide extremely detailed supervision. Although many of these representatives have, with years of practice, acquired considerable expertise and will give reliable advice, the principle involved in such collaboration is open to question and demands that the doctor exercises the utmost discretion. It is, of course, no defence in the event of difficulties for the doctor to claim that he was unaware of the status of his collaborator; it is his duty to ascertain this and this principle has been laid down in the law on many occasions.

We have laid considerable stress on the doctor's legal position in collaborating with others in the allergy team, because ultimately the doctor must be the one to take legal responsibility for the actions of all concerned. Nonetheless, the pressures on the time and skills of the doctor are considerable and sensible use of the skills available will always be helpful. To sum up, let it be said that running a successful team is not an attempt by the doctor to duck out of responsibilities because he is too busy; rather it is an attempt to use all the available skills to the best advantage of the patient. To collaborate successfully with other staff requires an understanding of their training and experience; a successful team operates on the basis of mutual trust and understanding which must never be abused. Viewed in this light, team work will yield results, in terms of both numbers seen and quality of work, far superior to those which are possible with a solo effort.

12

The Role of the Nurse in the Allergy Team

The care of the patient suffering symptoms of allergy is a team effort: no one career or discipline is in a position to identify and meet all of the needs which may arise. It is therefore essential that each team member identifies his or her own contribution and appreciates the contribution of others in order that successful team work based on mutual trust and understanding may operate to the best advantage of the patient. Nursing is one of the disciplines which is only as yet beginning to identify its own role and this chapter sets out to outline the contribution which nurses may make to the care of allergy patients.

Considerable interest has been aroused in the nursing profession by the use of the nursing process. This, simply stated, is a systematic and planned approach to the delivery of individualized nursing care. This problem-solving approach demands a thorough assessment of the patient; the identification of problems experienced; planned care appropriate to the identified problems; and a systematic evaluation of the care given. The patient is the central focus of such an approach to nursing. Whilst the medical diagnosis is of importance, it is only part of the information required to ensure appropriate nursing care. What is of greater significance is who and what the patient is and what effect his illness and its therapy has on his ability to function as an individual.

Allergy is a very common problem; a recent conservative estimate numbered 30% of the population of the UK as suffering allergy at some time in their life. Of course, not all will require medical care, but most will have to learn to live with their symptoms. The extent to which allergy interrupts normal functioning is a measure to the individual as to its severity. Similarly, the extent to which therapeutic measures enhance normal functioning will contribute towards continued compliance and success of treatment. It is in the field of assisting compliance that the nurse has a major contribution to make in the allergy team.

We have read in Chapter 11 that the primary role of the doctor in the team is to diagnose the type of allergy present and to prescribe and instigate a therapeutic regimen. The therapeutic regimen may comprise avoidance of the allergen, hyposensitization or palliative measures if the allergens are multiple and avoidance impracticable. The nurse may be called upon to assist with the diagnostic measures and also with the administration of treatments. However, this is not her only contribution. Although an important role and one which will be discussed later, this dependent role should not take precedence over the independent role of her own contribution as a nurse.

A well accepted definition of nursing by Virginia Henderson says: 'The unique function of the nurse is to assist the individual, sick or well, in the performance of those activities contributing to health or its recovering (or to peaceful death) that he would perform unaided if he had the necessary strength, will or knowledge, and to do this in such a way as to help him gain independence as rapidly as possible'. Let us consider this definition of nursing in the light of the role of the nurse in the allergy team.

The patients with whom the nurse will have contact are usually well, but frequently unable to function normally due to the symptoms their allergies produce. At first sight the preceding statement appears contradictory. How can someone be well yet unable to function normally? This is very much the paradox in which the allergy sufferer finds himself. To other people, friends, family and work-mates, the allergy sufferer is well apart from watery eyes, snuffly nose, perhaps an audible wheeze, but not ill. The perception of the individual sufferer may be quite different. What does one consider 'to function normally' to mean? Is it normal to cut the grass; to walk along country lanes; to live in the city/country; to seek employment; or to keep family pets? The list of activities is endless, but those in which the allergy sufferer may engage in may be severely curtailed if his symptoms are to be controlled.

So how can the nurse in the allergy team work towards the definition of nursing proposed by Henderson? Assisting the patient is a very broad expression and those who interpret it as simply doing things for patients, i.e. administering skin tests and injections etc., have a very limited perspective of their role. Assisting implies helping and there are many more meanings to this word than just doing things for patients. Guiding, teaching and counselling are all helping behaviours which comprise the meaning of assisting as used by Henderson. This type of assistance has far more to offer for the allergy patient, for ultimately it is the patient who must do for himself. The doing component of nursing care is only a very minor part of the function of nursing in the care of the allergy patient. The nurse can only help the patient to care for himself. This helping behaviour may simply be listening and advising about the difficulties encountered in enduring an allergen-restricted environment; suggesting and advising about other agencies which might be helpful, and monitoring and promoting inspiration in continuing the therapy prescribed. The relationship established between nurse and patient is of paramount importance, for it may well determine the extent to which the nurse may employ these helping behaviours in assisting the patient to function normally.

Having discussed the contribution of the nurse in the allergy team in general terms let us now examine the more particular aspects of her work with patients.

PATIENT ASSESSMENT

Assessment is a word with very broad meaning. In this instance it refers to the accumulation of information concerning the patient and his illness: his response to it and interruptions of daily living activities; the analysis of this information; and the statement of problems which present for him.

Several methods may be employed in assessing patients: observation, interviewing and reference to medical and/or nursing notes. Unfortunately, many nurses misinterpret the full meaning of patient assessment and for varied reasons rely solely on history-taking. However, this cannot provide a full understanding of the patient and his difficulties. How often do patients tell us what they think we want to hear? Our own observations of the patient provide considerable evidence to support or negate what the patient is telling us. For example, in response to the question 'How have you been since I last saw you?', the patient may well answer 'Oh, fine thank you': yet observation of the patient demonstrates runny eyes and nasal tone of voice. The nurse who takes the patient's answer at face value and fails to follow up her observation of cues may miss information pertinent to the continued care of the patient.

The example provided is very simple but demonstrates how errors of assessment can be made if only one method is employed. It is essential that information obtained from the patient by one method is corroborated by other methods in order to validate inferences and to arrive at correct identification of problems. Another example is taken from a consultation in an out-patient clinic.

John Smith, an 11-year-old boy, has a long history of inhalant allergy. Previous testing has demonstrated an allergy to *Aspergillus* sp. Rehousing in an old but centrally heated house and prophylactic use of bronchodilators has kept him moderately free of symptoms until recently, when bronchospasm and wheeze have returned necessitating several absences from school.

Examination by the doctor reveals moderately severe bronchospasm and the child looks obviously unwell. Questioning of both mother and child fails to demonstrate any change in therapy regimen and the cause of this exacerbation is unclear.

Throughout the interview, the clinic nurse has observed the mother's behaviour. She appears unusually 'ill at ease'. She sits on the edge of the chair; constantly fumbles with her house-keys; brushes away a younger sibling who attempts to cling to her; and frequently looks away from the doctor when answering his questions.

From this behaviour the nurse infers that Mrs Smith is

anxious and speaks aloud her inference: 'Mrs Smith, you seem very on edge—is there anything bothering you?' Mrs Smith replies that she is very worried. She has recently written a cheque for a large gas bill and does not have sufficient money in the bank to pay for it; her husband from whom she is separated fails to make maintenance payments and in order to economise she has turned off the central heating. The house is now cold and damp and John's chest problems started again shortly after the central heating was turned off.

In this example the nurse made an inference from the observations that Mrs Smith appeared anxious. However, observation alone could not explain the reason for the anxiety. Confirmation of the inference was sought by questioning Mrs Smith. The statement 'you seem very on edge' permitted Mrs Smith to agree or disagree with the nurse's inference, whilst the direct question 'is there anything bothering you?' provided Mrs Smith with the opportunity to disclose her anxieties if she so wished. In this instance Mrs Smith's response not only supported the inference of anxiety but also demonstrated its cause and in so doing provided information relevant to the exacerbation of John's illness.

These examples illustrate the necessity for a combination of methods to be employed in the assessment of patients. Emphasis has been placed on observation and interview but similarly reference to medical and nursing notes may provide supplementary or contradictory information. It is important that changed circumstances are noted or that previous experiences are taken into account when a full assessment of the patient is being made.

Patient history

Chapter 5 outlines the allergy history which the nurse may assist with or complete totally herself. The history form (pp. 45–47) requests detailed information pertaining to the allergy which will eventually assist the doctor in making a specific diagnosis. However, in addition, the topics listed may act as a prompt for the nurse to explore the patient's usual pattern of living and the extent to which it is interrupted by the presence of symptoms due to allergy.

The interview should be conducted in a relaxed manner. The skilful use of open-ended questions by the nurse should enable the patient to describe fully when and how his symptoms present and to what extent they interfere with his normal activities. The history form is pre-coded for easy reference. The experienced interviewer is able to tick the appropriate boxes during the interview and space is provided for particular observations and inferences to be recorded. The examples provided earlier illustrate the importance of the latter component of the patient history when analysing all of the information obtained to correctly identify patient problems.

It is emphasized that, although the format of the allergy history may give the appearance of a self-completing questionnaire, it should not be used in this manner. To do so could detract considerably from its value. Little or no background information would be available and, most important of all, the rapport between patient and nurse would be lost. The time spent in completing this form by means of interview is well spent for the relationship it enables is a valuable asset in the overall care of the patient.

The patient history and relevant observations provide considerable data from which the nurse may identify problems and the doctor suspect a diagnosis. But as noted earlier, these suspicions require confirmation and this is achieved by physical examination of the patient.

Physical examination

Physical examination of the patient is a controversial issue in nursing and one which will not be discussed at any length here. However, nurses working in allergy clinics frequently engage in a diagnostic component of physical examination.

The history provided by the patient may suggest hypersensitivity to one or more allergens, but objective confirmatory data must first be obtained before a final diagnosis can be made. This data is obtained by the use of skin testing and the nasal challenge test. (The reader is referred to Chapters 6 and 8 respectively for details of the methods employed in these tests and their interpretation.)

Although it is common practice for nurses to administer these tests, the type of test and strength of specific allergens used must be carefully prescribed by the doctor. Severe reactions and anaphylaxis are a remote possibility and therefore it is always advisable to have resuscitative measures readily available and adrenaline prepared for administration whenever these tests are undertaken.

Whilst experienced nurses may quickly acquire the knowledge and skills of interpreting the results of these tests, the final responsibility rests with the doctor who will be enabled to make a diagnosis.

The patient's history, observation and physical examination are the major components of information-gathering to which the nurse will make a specific contribution. Additional laboratory investigations are described in Chapters 7 and 8, but whilst the nurse may make reference to them, she is unlikely to participate in the laboratory tests themselves.

When all the information is available problem identification is possible. The medical diagnosis will, of course, be a focal point but it should be remembered that patient problems may be experienced in addition to or arising from the diagnosis and planned therapy. For this reason it is essential that nurses should contribute to problem identification and the planning of care.

PLANNING AND GIVING PATIENT CARE

The types of approaches to medical treatment are discussed in Chapters 9 and 10. It is not intended that these should be repeated here; the reader is advised to refer to the appropriate chapters. What is of particular relevance is their implication for nursing care. To refresh the reader's memory, medical treatment falls into three categories: allergen avoidance, hyposensitization and palliation using antihistamines and other drugs for prophylaxis. Various combinations of these regimens may be used.

The nursing implications also fall into three categories but of a very different nature: patient education, counselling and the administration of prescribed treatment. Let us consider each of these in turn.

Patient education

Successful alleviation of symptoms of allergy depends on the extent to which patients can organize their lives and cope with their prescribed treatment. The nurse's main caring responsibility is to help the patient care for himself and this can be achieved only if the patient knows why and what is to be done. Unless the patient understands why his symptoms present and what the basis of his treatment is, he is unlikely to cooperate fully with his treatment plan. This statement may perhaps seem nonsensical, for it might be assumed that because the patient has sought help he will automatically comply with the treatment regimen. However, this is untrue. Considerable research evidence demonstrates that patients do not always comply with treatment to the extent that nurses and doctors believe they do. This is particularly so when the treatment is long-term and when they are symptom-free.

Treatment for allergy is of necessity long-term and when successful the patient is symptom-free. The problem facing the nurse in caring for such patients is to maintain their motivation to comply with the planned treatment. This may be achieved by informing the patient of the reason for his treatment and how it works.

Simply telling the patient is not sufficient. It is very likely that the patient may not comprehend all that is told him or he may quickly forget the pertinent factors. Simple methods are available which ensure that the information retained by the patient is maximal. But before we engage in a discussion of teaching methods, it is essential that we start at the same point as the patient.

Determining what the patient knows is essential before planning what is to be taught. The approach to teaching an immunologist about his planned care would be very different to the approach taken with a manual worker. This is because their knowledge of the subject is very different. However, it is not always helpful to use examples of extremes: there are considerable differences in the knowledge possessed by patients and it is important that this should not be overlooked. At the same time, one ought not to assume knowledge that does not exist. Therefore, one must begin by assessing the level of knowledge the patient has of his allergy and its treatment. One may then explain in appropriate terms the type of allergy and how the symptoms it produces may be alleviated.

This verbal explanation should be supported by a *written* explanation outlining the major points. An example of such a written explanation may be found on p. 80. The pamphlet provides clear information and advice on the control of house dust mite and particularly important information is emphasized by the use of heavy type and capitals. This not only acts as an *aide memoire* for the patient but can also be used as incontrovertible evidence when helpful friends and neighbours offer conflicting advice!

In addition to written advice concerning allergen avoidance, a similar approach to the support of verbal explanation of self-administration of drugs and their possible side effects might be usefully employed.

Patient teaching is not something that is undertaken on one occasion only and is then completed. To bombard the patient with every detail possible on one occasion would only serve to overwhelm and confuse him. Information should be spaced and paced by the comprehension of the patient. This may, of course, present difficulties because of the spaced frequency of contact that the clinic nurse may have with the patient. However, this may be overcome by the inclusion of other people in the teaching programme. Patients may well have contact with other health workers in the course of their daily life, e.g. health visitors, school nurses, district nurses and occupational nurses. The clinic nurse may well be the instigator of the teaching programme but she does not necessarily have to be the sole teacher. In fact, these other nurses with whom the patient has contact may well be better placed to continue the teaching programme and motivation required, providing they are properly informed of what is planned.

Patient counselling

Counselling is one of the helping behaviours described at the beginning of this chapter. Some might argue that counselling is an important component of teaching and does not deserve consideration in its own right. However, the authors would disagree, for in this instance its remit is greater than simply in relation to the learning needs of the patient. Of course this is a large component but not the only one. Once a positive relationship has been established, patients frequently disclose difficulties and problems. The nurse will be able to assist with many of these problems but there will be those that fall outside her range of skills and knowledge. In these instances appropriate nursing action will be the referral of the patient to those agencies better able to be of assistance.

Problems and difficulties in compliance with the treatment will undoubtedly arise, particularly in relation to avoidance of allergens. For many reasons it may not prove possible to vacuum clean the house daily; to dispose of a much loved pet; to keep the house warm and dry—the list is endless. In these instances feelings of guilt may arise. These feelings of guilt, if left unexpressed, may give rise to tension within the home which is not conducive to normal family functioning. To be given the opportunity to express these feelings without fear of reproach but with understanding can do much to help patients and their families cope with the problem of allergy.

Administration of prescribed treatment

This is the aspect of nursing care which most readily comes to mind and for this reason it is discussed last. This is not to say that it is the least important, rather that for many it takes precedence over the other categories of nursing care which are of equal importance but which may, because of the pressure of time, be overlooked.

The prescribed treatment which the nurse may be called upon to administer is usually a course of hyposensitizing injections. These injections are given at weekly intervals over nine to twelve weeks and are administered deep subcutaneously. As discussed in Chapter 10, there is a risk of anaphylaxis following administration and for this reason resuscitative measures should be readily available. However, if a carefully prescribed dose is given correctly this should not happen and in the authors' experience has not yet been observed.

The administration of hyposensitizing injections is an extension of the nurse's usual role and as such she requires the security of a properly constructed policy agreed by her employing authority or employer which covers these duties. The policy should indicate what emergency drugs, if any, she may administer and such drugs must be provided and put out readily before the injection is given.

The administration of these injections is not solely a procedure to be completed in isolation; during the course of injections, the nurse should continue to assess her patient. Careful questioning regarding side effects should be undertaken at every stage of treatment and if any significant effects do occur then advice from the doctor should be sought. Usually, if a slight reaction occurs within eight hours of the injection, producing symptoms of allergy such as sneezing, runny nose or a minor wheeze, then the previous dose of hyposensitization is repeated. Because of the risk of anaphylaxis the decision is a medical one and should be referred to the doctor who should be on the premises and available whenever such injections are given.

There is of course a continuing need for patient education, not only in relation to the patients diagnosis and treatment as described above, but also for the wider issues of health education. The regular contact throughout the course of injections provides an opportunity for the nurse to explore and advise on health problems in addition to allergy.

The organization of the setting in which hyposensitization takes place is worth consideration. If the injections can be given during a session for allergy patients only, there are opportunities for self-help groups to form either spontaneously or specifically planned. Other patients can help each other with their problems. Useful tips on allergen avoidance, storage or drugs and mutual support from the realization that they are not alone with their problems nor abnormal can do much to help them live with their allergy.

The administration of prescribed treatment can therefore readily become a focal point for care and as such should be used for the broadest interpretation of nursing rather than simply the giving of an injection.

From the preceding discussion, it may be seen that although the three categories of nursing are distinct entities they are all interdependent, i.e. unless each component is practiced no single aspect of care will be successful in meeting the goals planned.

EVALUATION OF NURSING CARE

The framework advocated for a planned and systematic approach to nursing care requires that we evaluate the effectiveness of the care we provide for patients. This is something to which we have not given a great deal of attention in the past and consequently we do not have a vast range of evaluative methods available. However, as we become practised at setting realistic goals when planning patient care we will have something against which to measure our aim or the patient's performance. Setting realistic goals is the key to evaluating care, for they are the standards against which effectiveness of care can be measured. Targets may be set for each aspect of nursing care and the extent to which they have been achieved determined at each contact.

The methods employed in evaluation are not new but the same as those used in the stage of assessment. In fact, when evaluating care one is reassessing the problem and with it the extent to which the goals have been met.

However, when evaluating care given in respect of allergy, the achievement of these aims may not be evident for some time because of the seasonal or long-term nature of the problem. Nevertheless, this does not negate the need for setting goals and evaluating their achievement. Not all of those set will be of such a long-term nature. The understanding by the patient of his problem and the reasons for treatment needs to be evaluated sooner rather than later. Similarly the evaluation of advice given concerning difficulties arising from the treatment regimen.

Evaluation is an integral part of the problem solving approach to nursing; it might be claimed to be the most important component for it indicates the effectiveness or otherwise of all the efforts that have gone before. Such evaluation is onerous and therefore many nurses have opted to ignore it. However, unless evaluation is undertaken and the results recorded for reference, the work cannot be fully effective.

Nursing is a complex activity. In caring for the patient suffering from allergy the nurse cannot function alone, but she has a considerable contribution to make within the team. The nurses' contribution extends beyond the clinic into the home and working environment of the patient through the inclusion of nursing colleagues who comprise a wider team.

It should always be remembered that the most important member of the team is the patient, for it is he who ultimately controls the plan of care; it is he who decides whether or not to act upon the advice offered. The aim of nursing is to help the patient make the best possible use of the care offered so that he may eventually care for himself.

Sources of Help

BOOKS

Bencard, *Catalogue of Allergens*. Brentford.
Dome, *Catalogue of Allergens*. Slough.
Forsythe, E. (1975) *Asthma, Hay Fever and Other Allergies and How to Live With Them*. London: William Luscombe.
Garbe, D. R. & McDonnell, H. (1964) *Lung Function Testing.* Vitalograph.
Knight, A. (1981) *Asthma and Hay Fever*. Martin Dunitz.
Macauley, D. B. (1973) *Allergies.* Priory Press.
Mackarness, R. (1976) *Not All in the Mind*. London: Pan Books.
Mackarness, R. (1980) *Chemical Victims.* London: Pan Books.
Merrett, T. G. (1976) *Laboratory Assessment of the Allergic Patient*. Hounslow: Pharmacia.
Merck (1978) *Practical Allergy Using Norisen Extracts*. Alton: E. Merck.
Office of Health Economics (1976) *Asthma*. London: HMSO.
Rapp, D. J. & Frankland, A. W. (1976) *Allergies: Questions and Answers*. London: Heinemann Medical.

Most Medical or Nursing Libraries will also provide a list of journal articles on this subject.

ORGANIZATIONS

Action Against Allergy
43 The Downs, London SW20 8HG.
Asthma Society and Friends of the Asthma Research Council
12 Pembridge Square, London W24EH. Tel. 01 229 1142.
Medic-Alert Foundation
9 Hanover Street, London W1R 9HF.
Midlands Asthma and Allergy Research Association
12 Vernon Street, Derby. Tel. 0332 40366.
National Society for Research Into Allergy
PO Box 35, Hinckley, Leics.

Index

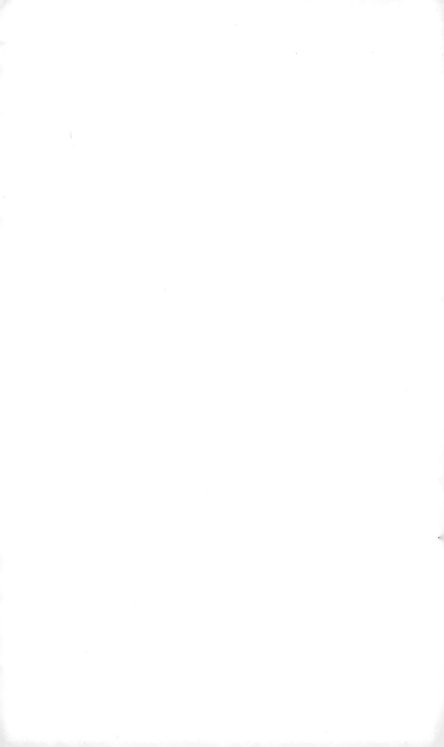